INNOVATIONS FOR TACKLING TUBERCULOSIS IN THE TIME OF COVID-19

PROCEEDINGS OF A WORKSHOP

Claire Biffl, Julie Liao, and Anna Nicholson, *Rapporteurs*

Forum on Microbial Threats

Board on Global Health

Health and Medicine Division

The National Academies of
SCIENCES • ENGINEERING • MEDICINE

THE NATIONAL ACADEMIES PRESS
Washington, DC
www.nap.edu

THE NATIONAL ACADEMIES PRESS   500 Fifth Street, NW   Washington, DC 20001

This activity was supported by a contract between the National Academy of Sciences and the U.S. Agency for International Development (10004113). Any opinions, findings, conclusions, or recommendations expressed in this publication do not necessarily reflect the views of any organization or agency that provided support for the project.

International Standard Book Number-13: 978-0-309-68642-6
International Standard Book Number-10: 0-309-68642-3
Digital Object Identifier: https://doi.org/10.17226/26530

This publication is available from the National Academies Press, 500 Fifth Street, NW, Keck 360, Washington, DC 20001; (800) 624-6242 or (202) 334-3313; http://www.nap.edu.

Copyright 2022 by the National Academy of Sciences. All rights reserved.

Printed in the United States of America

Suggested citation: National Academies of Sciences, Engineering, and Medicine. 2022. *Innovations for tackling tuberculosis in the time of COVID-19: Proceedings of a workshop.* Washington, DC: The National Academies Press. https://doi.org/10.17226/26530.

The National Academies of
SCIENCES · ENGINEERING · MEDICINE

The **National Academy of Sciences** was established in 1863 by an Act of Congress, signed by President Lincoln, as a private, nongovernmental institution to advise the nation on issues related to science and technology. Members are elected by their peers for outstanding contributions to research. Dr. Marcia McNutt is president.

The **National Academy of Engineering** was established in 1964 under the charter of the National Academy of Sciences to bring the practices of engineering to advising the nation. Members are elected by their peers for extraordinary contributions to engineering. Dr. John L. Anderson is president.

The **National Academy of Medicine** (formerly the Institute of Medicine) was established in 1970 under the charter of the National Academy of Sciences to advise the nation on medical and health issues. Members are elected by their peers for distinguished contributions to medicine and health. Dr. Victor J. Dzau is president.

The three Academies work together as the **National Academies of Sciences, Engineering, and Medicine** to provide independent, objective analysis and advice to the nation and conduct other activities to solve complex problems and inform public policy decisions. The National Academies also encourage education and research, recognize outstanding contributions to knowledge, and increase public understanding in matters of science, engineering, and medicine.

Learn more about the National Academies of Sciences, Engineering, and Medicine at **www.nationalacademies.org**.

The National Academies of
SCIENCES • ENGINEERING • MEDICINE

Consensus Study Reports published by the National Academies of Sciences, Engineering, and Medicine document the evidence-based consensus on the study's statement of task by an authoring committee of experts. Reports typically include findings, conclusions, and recommendations based on information gathered by the committee and the committee's deliberations. Each report has been subjected to a rigorous and independent peer-review process and it represents the position of the National Academies on the statement of task.

Proceedings published by the National Academies of Sciences, Engineering, and Medicine chronicle the presentations and discussions at a workshop, symposium, or other event convened by the National Academies. The statements and opinions contained in proceedings are those of the participants and are not endorsed by other participants, the planning committee, or the National Academies.

For information about other products and activities of the National Academies, please visit www.nationalacademies.org/about/whatwedo.

COMMITTEE ON INNOVATIONS FOR TACKLING TUBERCULOSIS IN THE TIME OF COVID-19: A TWO-PART WORKSHOP[1]

GAIL H. CASSELL (*Co-Chair*), Senior Lecturer on Global Health and Social Medicine, Harvard Medical School
KENNETH G. CASTRO (*Co-Chair*), Professor of Global Health, Epidemiology, and Infectious Diseases, Rollins School of Public Health and School of Medicine, Emory University
EMILY ABRAHAM, Director, External Affairs and Policy, Global Public Health at Johnson & Johnson
ANDREW CLEMENTS, Senior Technical Advisor, Emerging Threats Division, U.S. Agency for International Development
LUCICA DITIU, Executive Director, Stop TB Partnership, United Nations Office for Project Services
MARCOS A. ESPINAL, Director, Communicable Diseases and Environmental Determinants of Health, Pan American Health Organization
HAMIDAH HUSSAIN, Director, IRD Global
TEREZA KASAEVA, Director, Global Tuberculosis Programme, World Health Organization
KENT E. KESTER, Vice President and Head, Translational Science and Biomarkers, Sanofi Pasteur
MONIQUE K. MANSOURA, Executive Director, Global Health Security and Biotechnology, MITRE
PETER SANDS, Executive Director, The Global Fund to Fight AIDS, Tuberculosis and Malaria
CHARLES WELLS, Head of Therapeutics Development, Bill & Melinda Gates Medical Research Institute

National Academies Staff

JULIE LIAO, Director, Forum on Microbial Threats
ELIZABETH ASHBY, Associate Program Officer
CHARLES MINICUCCI, Research Assistant
CLAIRE BIFFL, Research Assistant
JULIE PAVLIN, Senior Board Director

---

[1] The planning committee's role was limited to planning the workshop, and the Proceedings of a Workshop was prepared by the workshop rapporteurs as a factual summary of what occurred at the workshop. Statements, recommendations, and opinions expressed are those of individual presenters and participants and are not necessarily endorsed or verified by the National Academies of Sciences, Engineering, and Medicine, and they should not be construed as reflecting any group consensus.

FORUM ON MICROBIAL THREATS[1]

PETER DASZAK (*Chair*), President, EcoHealth Alliance
KENT E. KESTER (*Vice Chair*), Vice President and Head, Translational Science and Biomarkers, Sanofi Pasteur
RIMA F. KHABBAZ (*Vice Chair*), Director, National Center for Emerging Zoonotic Infectious Diseases, U.S. Centers for Disease Control and Prevention
EMILY ABRAHAM, Director, External Affairs and Policy, Global Public Health at Johnson & Johnson
KEVIN ANDERSON, Senior Program Manager, Science and Technology Directorate, U.S. Department of Homeland Security
CRISTINA CASSETTI, Deputy Division Director, Division of Microbiology and Infectious Diseases, National Institute of Allergy and Infectious Diseases
ANDREW CLEMENTS, Senior Technical Advisor, Emerging Threats Division, U.S. Agency for International Development
SCOTT F. DOWELL, Deputy Director for Surveillance and Epidemiology, Bill & Melinda Gates Foundation
MARCOS A. ESPINAL, Director, Communicable Diseases and Environmental Determinants of Health, Pan American Health Organization
EVA HARRIS, Professor, Division of Infectious Diseases and Vaccinology; Director, Center for Global Public Health, University of California, Berkeley School of Public Health
ELIZABETH D. HERMSEN, Head, Global Antimicrobial Stewardship and Health Equity in Infectious Diseases, Merck & Co., Inc.
CHRISTOPHER R. HOUCHENS, Director, Division of Chemical, Biological, Radiological and Nuclear Countermeasures, Biomedical Advanced Research and Development Authority
CHANDY C. JOHN, Director, Ryan White Center for Pediatric Infectious Disease and Global Health, Indiana University School of Medicine and Riley Hospital for Children at IU Health
MARK G. KORTEPETER, Vice President for Research, Professor of Preventive Medicine and Medicine, Uniformed Services University of the Health Sciences

---

[1] The National Academies of Sciences, Engineering, and Medicine's forums and roundtables do not issue, review, or approve individual documents. The responsibility for the published Proceedings of a Workshop rests with the workshop rapporteurs and the institution.

MICHAEL MAIR, Acting Assistant Commissioner for Counterterrorism Policy; Acting Director, Office of the Chief Scientist, U.S. Food and Drug Administration
JONNA A. K. MAZET, Vice Provost—Grand Challenges; Chancellor's Leadership Professor of Epidemiology & Disease Ecology, University of California, Davis
VICTORIA McGOVERN, Senior Program Officer, Burroughs Wellcome Fund
SALLY A. MILLER, Distinguished Professor of Food, Agricultural and Environmental Sciences in Plant Pathology, The Ohio State University, College of Food, Agriculture, and Environmental Sciences
SUERIE MOON, Director of Research, Global Health Centre; Visiting Lecturer, Graduate Institute of International and Development Studies; Adjunct Lecturer, Harvard T.H. Chan School of Public Health
RAFAEL OBREGON, Country Representative, UNICEF Paraguay
KUMANAN RASANATHAN, Unit Head for Equity and Health, Department of Social Determinants of Health, World Health Organization
GARY A. ROSELLE, Executive Director, National Infectious Disease Services Program, Veterans Health Administration, U.S. Department of Veterans Affairs
PETER A. SANDS, Executive Director, The Global Fund to Fight AIDS, Tuberculosis & Malaria
THOMAS W. SCOTT, Distinguished Professor, Department of Entomology and Nematology, University of California, Davis
MATTHEW ZAHN, Deputy Health Officer, Orange County Health Care Agency

National Academies of Sciences, Engineering, and Medicine Staff

JULIE LIAO, Director, Forum on Microbial Threats
ELIZABETH ASHBY, Associate Program Officer
CHARLES MINICUCCI, Research Assistant (*until September 2021*)
CLAIRE BIFFL, Research Assistant
JUSTIN HAMMERBERG, Senior Program Assistant (*from January 2022*)
JULIE PAVLIN, Senior Board Director

Reviewers

This Proceedings of a Workshop was reviewed in draft form by individuals chosen for their diverse perspectives and technical expertise. The purpose of this independent review is to provide candid and critical comments that will assist the National Academies of Sciences, Engineering, and Medicine in making each published proceedings as sound as possible and to ensure that it meets the institutional standards for quality, objectivity, evidence, and responsiveness to the charge. The review comments and draft manuscript remain confidential to protect the integrity of the process.

We thank the following individuals for their review of this proceedings:

KUNCHOK DORJEE, Johns Hopkins University
ANNA MARIA MANDALAKAS, Baylor College of Medicine
ELTONY MUGOMERI, Africa University

Although the reviewers listed above provided many constructive comments and suggestions, they were not asked to endorse the content of this proceedings nor did they see the final draft before its release. The review of this proceedings was overseen by **ANN M. ARVIN,** Stanford University. She was responsible for making certain that an independent examination of this proceedings was carried out in accordance with the standards of the National Academies and that all review comments were carefully considered. Responsibility for the final content rests entirely with the rapporteurs and the National Academies.

Acknowledgments

The workshop summarized in this proceedings is the product of many valuable contributions. Special thanks go to the presenters and discussants who gave generously of their time and expertise to make the event possible.

In memory of Dr. Hamidah Hussain.

Contents

ACRONYMS AND ABBREVIATIONS   xvii

1   **INTRODUCTION**   1
     Workshop Objectives, 2
     Organization of the Proceedings of the Workshop, 3

2   **CURRENT TOOLS AND CHALLENGES**   5
     Leadership from Public Health Workers in Ending
       Tuberculosis—Past and Present, 6
     Progress Toward Global Tuberculosis Elimination Goals and
       Opportunities for Moving Forward, 8
     Challenges and Innovations, 12
     New Technologies and Remaining Gaps in Tuberculosis
       Diagnostics, 14
     Improving Treatment Regimens and Vaccine Development, 17
     Collective Social Value of Infectious Disease Interventions, 20
     Discussion, 23

3   **DETECTION**   29
     USAID's Commitment to Addressing Tuberculosis Worldwide, 30
     Building a Tuberculosis-Free World: Progress Update, 32
     Realities of Multidrug-Resistant Tuberculosis, 37
     Rapid Acceleration of Diagnostics Technology:
       COVID-19 Pandemic Experience, 41
     Advances in Tuberculosis Diagnostics, 47

Improving Adherence, Infection Control Capacities, and
　　Cost-Effectiveness, 51

4　VACCINES AND THERAPEUTICS　　　　　　　　　　　　73
　　Existing Tools and New Technologies, 74
　　Transforming Treatment Options, 88
　　Reflections and Discussion on Critical Elements
　　　　for Implementation, 111
　　Discussion, 117

5　FINANCING, AMBITION, AND PREPAREDNESS　　　　　123
　　A Place for Tuberculosis in the Pandemic Preparedness
　　　　Agenda, 125
　　Achieving Synergy in Global Health Security Preparedness
　　　　Against Respiratory Pathogens, 132
　　Making the Case for Financing Tuberculosis Elimination, 142
　　Final Comments, 153

APPENDIXES
A　REFERENCES　　　　　　　　　　　　　　　　　　　　155
B　WORKSHOP STATEMENT OF TASK　　　　　　　　　　165
C　WORKSHOP AGENDA　　　　　　　　　　　　　　　　167

Boxes, Figures, and Table

BOXES

2-1 Progress in Reducing the Global Tuberculosis Burden, 9
2-2 Challenges and Opportunities in Advancing Tuberculosis Diagnostics, 17

3-1 Investment Priorities for Ending Tuberculosis, 34
3-2 Point-of-Care Technologies Research Network, 42
3-3 Research Priorities in the Cascade of Tuberculosis Prevention, 68

4-1 Overview of Lessons Learned from TBTC Study 31/A5349, 94
4-2 Lessons Learned from the Rollout of Bedaquiline in South Africa, 101
4-3 Performance-Based Monitoring and Evaluation Framework: Core Indicators, 114

FIGURES

3-1 Progress toward 2018–2022 global targets for the number of people treated for tuberculosis, 40
3-2 Preparedness framework, 59

4-1 Bacillus Calmette–Guérin vaccination policies worldwide, 75
4-2 Potential uses of a tuberculosis vaccine, 79

4-3 Primary efficacy results for Tuberculosis Trials Consortium Study 31/AIDS Clinical Trials Group A5349, 90

4-4 USAID's Performance-Based Monitoring and Evaluation Framework, 113

TABLE

4-1 Optimal Pan-Tuberculosis Target Regimen Profile, 104

Acronyms and Abbreviations

AMR	antimicrobial resistance
AU	Africa University
BARDA	Biomedical Advanced Research and Development Authority
BCG	Bacillus Calmette-Guérin
BMGF	Bill and Melinda Gates Foundation
CEPI	Coalition for Epidemic Preparedness Innovations
CHW	community health worker
DALY	disability-adjusted life year
DARPA	Defense Advanced Research Projects Agency
DAT	digital adherence technology
DOTS	directly observed treatment, short-course
DR TB	drug-resistant tuberculosis
DS TB	drug-susceptible tuberculosis
ECG	electrocardiogram
FDA	U.S. Food and Drug Administration
GDP	gross domestic product
HIV	human immunodeficiency virus

HLIP	High-Level Independent Panel
HR	human resources
ICEC	International Cancer Expert Corps
IFI	international financial institutions
IGRA	interferon gamma release assay
IHR	International Health Regulations
IMF	International Monetary Fund
IMI	Innovative Medicines Initiative
IRB	institutional review board
IRD	Interactive Research and Development
J&J	Johnson and Johnson
LMIC	low- and middle-income country
MDG	Millennium Development Goal
MDR TB	multidrug resistant tuberculosis
mRNA	messenger RNA
NGO	nongovernmental organization
NHP	nonhuman primate
NIH	National Institutes of Health
PAN-TB	Project to Accelerate New Treatments for Tuberculosis
PCR	polymerase chain reaction
PEPFAR	President's Emergency Plan for AIDS Relief
POC	point-of-care
POCTRN	Point-of-Care Technologies Research Network
PPR	pandemic preparedness and response
R&D	research and development
ROI	return on investment
RR TB	rifampicin-resistant tuberculosis
SDG	Sustainable Development Goal
TB	tuberculosis
TBDA	TB Drug Accelerator
TPT	tuberculosis preventive therapy
TRP	target regimen profile
TST	tuberculin or tuberculosis skin test

UHC	universal health care
UN	United Nations
UNHLM	United Nations High-Level Meeting
USAID	United States Agency for International Development
WHO	World Health Organization
XDR TB	extensively drug-resistant tuberculosis

1

Introduction

Despite being preventable and curable since the middle of the twentieth century, tuberculosis (TB) has long persisted as the world's deadliest infectious disease, with the communities most devastated by TB among the poorest and most vulnerable in the world. Each year, approximately 10 million new people become sick with TB—it is estimated that an additional 3 million people go undiagnosed—and 1.4 million people die of the disease (WHO, 2020). Only about half of people with TB receive successful treatment each year. As the global threat of antimicrobial resistance continues to escalate, so do cases of drug-resistant TB, or TB that is resistant to various antibiotics that constitute standard treatment regimens. In 2020, more than 500,000 people became ill with drug-resistant TB, yet only one in three had access to treatment (WHO, 2021d).

Since TB was declared a global health emergency by the World Health Organization (WHO) in 1993, momentum has been building toward eliminating TB across the world through the development and implementation of more effective strategies to detect and diagnose people with TB, support them throughout treatment, and prevent them from spreading TB within their families and communities. Although these efforts have had a significant effect on the global disease burden, much work remains to close critical gaps in detection, diagnosis, treatment, and prevention of TB in order to avert unnecessary suffering and death caused by the disease.

Unfortunately, COVID-19 and its mitigation efforts have taken a destructive toll on countries with the highest burden of TB disease and have diverted attention and resources from the global TB response, threatening to reverse years of progress toward eliminating the disease. Alarmingly, the majority of countries across the world have reported decreases in both the numbers of people diagnosed with TB and the number of patients receiving treatment during the COVID-19 pandemic (Stop TB Partnership, 2021). Recent modeling exercises estimate that the initial effect in 2020 of the COVID-19 pandemic will result in an additional 1.4 million TB deaths between 2020 and 2025 (Stop TB Partnership, 2020). WHO (2021b) has also estimated that rates of TB will be higher in 2021 than in recent years, while worldwide TB case notifications will decrease by 21 percent and an additional 500,000 deaths will occur between 2019 and 2020.[1]

Ambitious global targets for TB elimination have been established by the United Nations High-Level Meeting (UNHLM) on Tuberculosis (UN, 2018), which set targets for 2022, and WHO's End TB Strategy, which set targets for 2030 (WHO, 2015). Even prior to the COVID-19 pandemic, the rate of progress in global TB control had stagnated and the pace was insufficient to achieve those goals without urgent collective action by the international TB control community. In the midst of the COVID-19 pandemic, those efforts will need to be redoubled to avoid losing ground in the fight against TB and to foster a renewed global commitment to tackling the disease.

WORKSHOP OBJECTIVES

On July 22, 2021, and September 14–16, 2021, a planning committee under the auspices of the Forum on Microbial Threats at the National Academies of Sciences, Engineering, and Medicine held a two-part virtual workshop titled Innovations for Tackling Tuberculosis in the Time of COVID-19.[2] The aims of the workshop were (1) to evaluate the current status of TB elimination, (2) to assess the effects of the COVID-19 pandemic on the global fight against TB, and (3) to examine technical and strategic innovations that could be used to meet the UNHLM targets in 2022 and WHO's End TB Strategy targets by 2030. The virtual workshop featured invited presentations and discussions to consider the following:[3]

---

[1] TB is a notifiable disease in many countries. This means providers are required to report diagnosed TB cases to relevant health authorities, and these data are ultimately shared with WHO. Reporting requirements are not uniform across all countries, and the End TB Strategy has called for enforcing current notification requirements. For more information see Uplekar et al., 2016, and WHO, 2015.

[2] The planning committee's role was limited to planning the workshop, and the Proceedings of a Workshop was prepared by the workshop rapporteurs as a factual summary of what occurred at the workshop. Statements, recommendations, and opinions expressed are those of individual presenters and participants and are not necessarily endorsed or verified by the National Academies of Sciences, Engineering, and Medicine, and they should not be construed as reflecting any group consensus.

[3] The list of references is found in Appendix A. The full statement of task is in Appendix B, and the workshop agenda is available in Appendix C.

- How can we accelerate the development of affordable point-of-care tests for TB? What barriers or challenges have prevented the development of accessible point-of-care tests for TB in low- and middle-income countries?
- Improvements in the usual care for TB: Can we achieve a 2-week, nontoxic treatment for drug-sensitive and drug-resistant TB?
- How can we rapidly use the TB platform, such as contact investigation, in low- and middle-income countries to address COVID-19 and other airborne infections to prevent future pandemics?
- How can we ensure increased and sustained commitments to reach the UNHLM?

ORGANIZATION OF THE PROCEEDINGS OF THE WORKSHOP

In accordance with the policies of the National Academies, the workshop did not attempt to establish any conclusions or recommendations about needs and future directions, focusing instead on information presented, questions raised, and improvements suggested by individual workshop participants. Chapter 2 summarizes the first part of the workshop, which focused on current tools and challenges related to tackling tuberculosis in the time of COVID-19. Chapter 3 explores the state of TB detection worldwide and the progress underway to improve case finding, diagnostics, and notification. Chapter 4 examines advancements in TB vaccines and therapeutics. Chapter 5 addresses ways to bolster financing, ambition, and preparedness in strategies to eliminate TB in a global context that has been dramatically changed by the COVID-19 pandemic.

2

Current Tools and Challenges

Part 1 of the workshop series, which focused on current tools and challenges related to tackling tuberculosis during the COVID-19 pandemic, was moderated by Kenneth Castro, professor of global health, epidemiology, and infectious diseases at Emory University, and Gail Cassell, senior lecturer on global health and social medicine at Harvard Medical School. The workshop featured three opening addresses on the current status and urgency of ending TB around the world. Jim Yong Kim, vice president and partner at Global Infrastructure Partners, highlighted the critical role of leadership and the value of strong community-based public health systems. Salmaan Keshavjee, director of the Harvard Medical School Center for Global Health Delivery and chair of the Steering Committee of the Zero TB Initiative, discussed progress toward global TB elimination and presented a comprehensive epidemic control strategy with potential to bolster those efforts. Eric Rubin, editor-in-chief of the *New England Journal of Medicine*, focused on innovations and translatable lessons from the COVID-19 pandemic regarding diagnostics, therapeutics, and vaccines for TB.

The subsequent session explored challenges and innovations in efforts to eliminate TB. Soumya Swaminathan, chief scientist of the World Health Organization (WHO), described new technologies and remaining gaps in TB diagnostics. Emilio Emini, director of the human immunodeficiency virus (HIV) and TB program at the Bill and Melinda Gates Foundation (BMGF),[1]

---

[1] Since the time of the workshop in July 2021, Emini transitioned to a new role as the chief executive officer at the Bill & Melinda Gates Medical Research Institute.

explored challenges and opportunities in developing improved TB therapeutics and vaccines. Kevin Outterson, co-director of the Boston University Health Law Program and the founding executive director of the Combating Antibiotic-Resistant Bacteria Biopharmaceutical Accelerator (CARB-X),[2] delved into the collective social value of infectious disease interventions.

LEADERSHIP FROM PUBLIC HEALTH WORKERS IN ENDING TUBERCULOSIS—PAST AND PRESENT

Presented by Jim Yong Kim, Global Infrastructure Partners

Kim opened by describing the value of strong community-based public health systems and the critical role of leadership in driving efforts to eliminate TB. To reflect on ways the approach to TB specifically—and to global health more broadly—have both changed and remained constant over the past 2 decades, he began by recounting his experience working in Peru with Partners In Health in the 1990s.[3] His team identified 50 cases of multi-drug resistant (MDR) TB in a squatters' settlement, and proposed to the country's National TB Program that those people should be treated, both for the patients' direct benefit and to halt future transmission to other members of the community. Kim's team was surprised to encounter strong opposition from both the National TB Program leader and from WHO. At the time, Kim said, WHO was actively discouraging the treatment of MDR TB in developing countries owing to concerns that it would draw attention away from the standard, "directly observed treatment, short-course" (DOTS) program,[4] which had been a transformative innovation in TB control (Partners In Health, 2006). Kim and his team eventually persuaded the National TB Program to explore the potential benefits of treating people with MDR TB, and WHO has since changed its policy. However, the team later faced similar resistance when advocating to the global health community for the treatment of HIV infections in some low- and middle-income countries (LMICs) in Africa, which was presumed to be infeasible to implement. That barrier was also surmounted, and today more than 20 million people are receiving HIV treatment in LMICs in Africa.

---

[2] For more information on CARB-X, visit https://carb-x.org (accessed August 18 2021).

[3] More information about Partners in Health is available at https://www.pih.org (accessed December 15, 2021).

[4] Directly observed treatment, short-course (DOTS) is an approach to managing TB whereby patients consume their doses of antituberculosis drugs under the supervision of a health care worker to ensure that the patient receives the appropriate medication at the right doses and intervals (Otu, 2013). WHO began promoting the DOTS approach in 1993, after the declaration of TB as a global health emergency, and it has had broad uptake worldwide.

This pattern of resistance has continued to the present day, Kim noted. When COVID-19 began to spread in early 2020, he was told by leaders in the U.S. public health community that it was "too late or too complicated" to conduct widespread contact tracing and stop the spread in the United States; others recommended waiting for herd immunity to develop. Kim countered that view by highlighting the substantial pandemic-related economic loss due to COVID-19, estimated at $16 trillion by Cutler and Summers (2020), with $7.6 trillion in lost economic output. Cutler and Summers contended that those potential losses serve as reasonable justification for spending $100 billion per year to build U.S. public health system capacities, including testing and contact-tracing systems. Kim reaffirmed that mitigating MDR TB will require vaccines, therapeutics, and diagnostics. Further, he said that a solid public health foundation is a critical element of the task. Those in the TB community have a wealth of experience in building that ground game, Kim said, and he encouraged them to take central leadership roles in establishing public health systems that can stop TB, COVID-19, and other infectious disease threats yet to come. Kim posited that the COVID-19 pandemic will catalyze more funding support to counter a range of infectious diseases, but that "leaders in the community must put forth a brilliant, compelling, integrated vision of what these new public health systems will look like" in order to optimize these resources.

Cassell asked how development banks might help accomplish that goal. Kim replied that his former colleagues at the World Bank are eager to support countries that are seeking to develop public health systems that are fully equipped for a range of infectious and noninfectious health threats. Development banks are looking for models of more horizontal health systems—such as programs delivered by community health workers (CHWs)—that are broader in scope and could therefore have a higher return on investment than vertical programs (e.g., TB-only projects). He emphasized that the TB community is uniquely qualified to lead in these horizontal programs by drawing upon decades of experience in implementing components of DOTS that could be applied to other efforts: finding cases, investigating contacts, promoting treatment adherence, and implementing infection control and prevention measures. For example, Kim noted, Partners in Health developed a program in Massachusetts to highlight the host of benefits of CHW engagement that evolved from early contact-tracing efforts:

- Close proximity to and relationships with community members, which contributed to the success of various health care interventions (e.g., supporting patients in isolation, conducting vaccination outreach, delivering treatments);
- Increased ability to reach isolated communities;

- Horizontal integration of multiple disease programs to appeal to global funders; and
- Economic stimulus to enable individuals who might otherwise be unemployed during a disease outbreak to remain in the workforce, with their salaries returned to the local economy through spending.

Cassell relayed a question about the relationship between metrics to assess global health preparedness and the access and sustainability of financing for such efforts. Kim highlighted the fundamental role of leadership in ensuring the success of multilateral systems and noted that the bottleneck to be addressed is not a lack of money—as evidenced by the economic stimulus measures taken by the United States and other countries—but the lack of alignment and agreement across the leadership of the multilateral organizations. Discord among leaders or a change in leadership can render current systems—including metrics—and available funding both irrelevant and ineffectual. Thus, the challenge is to use the attention and new sources of capital associated with the COVID-19 pandemic to build better systems, including metrics, and establish strong baseline capacities that are resilient to changes in leadership.

PROGRESS TOWARD GLOBAL TUBERCULOSIS ELIMINATION GOALS AND OPPORTUNITIES FOR MOVING FORWARD

Presented by Salmaan Keshavjee, Harvard Medical School

Keshavjee discussed the status of efforts to eliminate TB in the time of COVID-19 and opportunities to move those efforts forward. According to WHO's Global Tuberculosis Reports for 2019 and 2020, roughly 10 million people became ill and were diagnosed with TB each year, but there were an estimated additional 3 million undiagnosed or unreported TB cases. Although TB has been curable since the 1940s, only 56 percent of total TB treatments in 2019 and 2020 were successful, and an estimated 1.5 million people died from TB in each of those years—including more than 250,000 people living with HIV annually. Around the world, about 500,000 new people fell ill in 2019 and 2020 with drug-resistant (DR) TB, only one in three had access to treatment, and only one in five were cured (WHO, 2019, 2020).

Keshavjee provided an overview of progress toward global TB elimination targets set forth by WHO and the United Nations High-Level Meeting (UNHLM) on Tuberculosis (UN, 2018) to emphasize that the TB community fell dramatically short of reaching the End TB Strategy goals for 2015–2020 and that efforts were insufficient to meet the UNHLM goals for 2018–2020 (Box 2-1). This glacial pace of progress over the past decade extends across epidemiological trends for both drug-sensitive (or drug-susceptible, DS)

> **BOX 2-1**
> **Progress in Reducing the Global Tuberculosis Burden**
>
> **Progress toward the goals set by the End TB Strategy**
>
> - Incidence rate: goal of 20 percent reduction between 2015–2020, achieved 9 percent
> - Number of deaths: goal of 35 percent reduction between 2015–2020, achieved 14 percent
> - Share of patients facing catastrophic treatment costs: goal of 100 percent reduction by 2020, achieved a 49 percent reduction
>
> **Progress toward the goals set by the United Nations High-Level Meeting for 2018–2022**
>
> - TB treatment: goal of 40 million, treated 14.1 million (35 percent) in 2018 and 2019
> - TB preventive treatment: goal of 30 million, treated 6.3 million (21 percent) in 2018 and 2019
> - TB preventive treatment in people living with HIV: goal of 6.0 million, reached 88 percent of goal in 2018 and 2019
> - TB preventive treatment in household contacts under the age of 5: goal of 4.0 million, reached 20 percent of goal in 2018 and 2019
> - TB preventive treatment in household contacts older than the age of 5: goal of 20 million, reached less than 1 percent in 2018 and 2019
> - TB treatment in children: goal of 3.5 million, treated 1.04 million (30 percent) in 2018 and 2019
> - Treatment for MDR or rifampicin-resistant (RR) TB: goal of 1.5 million but treated approximately 20 percent of goal in 2018 and 2019
> - Treatment of MDR or RR TB in children: goal of 115,000, treated approximately 8 percent of goal in 2018 and 2019
>
> SOURCES: Presented by Salmaan Keshavjee on July 22, 2021; WHO, 2020.

TB and DR TB, he noted. One of the goals set by the End TB Strategy is to achieve a 20 percent reduction in TB incidence between 2015 and 2020. Prior to the COVID-19 pandemic, only a 9 percent reduction in global TB incidence rate was reported. Between 2006 and 2016, the annualized incidence rate for DS TB and DR TB saw only small declines of 1.3 percent and 2.1 percent, respectively (Kyu et al., 2018). During the same period, the annualized incidence rate for extensively drug-resistant (XDR) TB increased by 7.9 percent. Moreover, 70 percent of the officers from Global Fund implementing countries reported a decrease in the number of TB patients receiving treatment during COVID-19, with 88 percent reporting a reduction of TB case notification (Stop TB Partnership, 2021). Even more worrisome, noted

Keshavjee, is that WHO has estimated that more people will develop the disease in 2021, creating the potential for 1.8 million deaths attributable to TB. Keshavjee emphasized that the current rate of treatment being delivered is low, particularly in high-burden countries.

Potential Pathway to the Elimination of Tuberculosis: Search-Treat-Prevent Strategy

Despite acknowledging these concerning trends and stagnated progress toward global TB control targets, Keshavjee was resolute in his belief that TB elimination is possible and can be achieved by implementing a comprehensive epidemic control strategy—"search-treat-prevent"—that has existed since the 1960s but has yet to be implemented on a global scale, particularly in high-burden LMICs. Beyond addressing the global burden of TB, the strategy could also serve as a platform for controlling other infectious disease threats such as COVID-19. Knowledge and practice of each component in the search-treat-prevent strategy date back to the beginning and middle of the twentieth century, said Keshavjee. He explained how each component of the three-pronged strategy can be applied to TB control.

The first prong is to search for people with TB infection and disease through active case finding around small numbers of cases or community screening in epidemic settings. It has been established since the early twentieth century that early case detection leads to lower mortality, even before TB treatments were available (Golub et al., 2005). Today, active case finding using a sensitive diagnostic remains a critical tool for finding active cases and stopping transmission of TB. Keshavjee noted that mobile X-ray has been the primary diagnostic modality since the last century. Today, a range of other diagnostic tools is available including artificial intelligence (AI)-supported X-ray screening, culture testing, and rapid molecular testing tools to confirm TB infection, disease, and drug susceptibility. However, these tools are not being deployed everywhere they could be, and they are often entirely unavailable in high-burden TB countries, thus contributing to the lack of progress in driving down TB rates worldwide, Keshavjee added.

The second prong is to treat TB disease by administering the correct medicines with the fewest side effects over the shortest possible treatment period. As the global TB statistics demonstrate, the TB control community has fallen significantly short of treating the numbers of TB patients needed to stop community transmission of the disease and avert death and suffering. However, one opportunity to address this treatment gap is the availability of new drug regimens that are less burdensome to patients—such as short-course DS TB regimens that reduce treatment time from 6 to 4 months and all-oral DR TB regimens. The provision of patient supports, such as food and cash transfers and other economics-based behavior innovations, can also encourage treatment completion.

The third prong aims to prevent infections from turning into active disease as well as stop the transmission of TB infections. One preventive approach to infection and transmission control that has long been discussed for TB, but has recently risen to prominence during the COVID-19 pandemic, involves the use of respirators, ventilation, and upper-room ultraviolet germicidal lighting. However, these have been difficult to roll out in resource-limited settings because of a lack of focus on implementing engineering controls for preventing TB transmission in congregate settings.

It has been established since the 1950s that active case finding, treatment of all forms of TB disease, and treatment of TB infection using isoniazid prophylaxis could virtually eliminate household and community TB transmission (Kaplan et al., 1972). Between 5 and 10 percent of individuals infected will develop TB disease during their lifetime; of these, about 50 percent will develop TB within 2 years of infection (CDC, 2014). Thus, based on current TB incidence statistics, tens of million contacts should receive prophylactic treatment each year worldwide. He acknowledged that this number may seem daunting, but pointed out that it is logistically feasible to reach and treat the close contacts of patients who are already receiving treatment for active TB. He added that the conceptualization of latent versus clinically active TB is a false binary (Cadena et al., 2016); rather, there is a continuum between infection and disease. "Sometimes people that don't really appear to have clinically active disease are actually shedding bugs," he said. Keshavjee highlighted new tools and opportunities that have recently emerged or been expanded in the prevention domain, such as new short-course preventive treatment regimens for DS TB (e.g., 1 month of isoniazid or rifapentine, or 3 months of once weekly isoniazid and rifapentine) and new treatment regimens for MDR and XDR TB (e.g., bedaquiline, ongoing clinical trial using levofloxacin). Opportunities also exist to use existing treatment regimens to increase coverage of preventive therapy, he added.

The search-treat-prevent strategy has been effectively applied to accelerate TB elimination in settings around the world since the 1950s, notably in Alaska and New York City in the United States; Tomsk, the Russian Federation; and Karachi, Pakistan (Keshavjee et al., 2008). Keshavjee called for renewed commitment to build on those past success in designing and implementing TB elimination initiatives that are comprehensive, simultaneous, and based on efficacious tools and strategies as the standard of care for TB. Moreover, he suggested that donor countries insist that global development funders support programs that are comprehensive and designed to meet global TB elimination targets, rather than fund programs that do not perform to their optimal potential despite continued investment.

Building a Versatile Platform for Community-Based Care Delivery

Keshavjee explained how a community-based TB care delivery platform could evolve into a platform that supports the treatment and prevention of a wide range of diseases—including endemic infectious diseases, noncommunicable diseases (e.g., diabetes, heart disease, and mental illness), and emerging infectious diseases such as COVID-19—by extending the capabilities and deepening the reach of clinics into communities. He added that the present moment offers an opportunity to shift the global TB control paradigm in a way that will strengthen global biosecurity. Establishing comprehensive TB control systems is synergistic with efforts to bolster global biosecurity and pandemic preparedness because the capacities required for TB control are broadly applicable to many different biosecurity-related health care priorities. However, catalytic investment through global funding mechanisms and bilateral programs is needed to support communities and programs in implementing the comprehensive search-treat-prevent strategy worldwide.

Keshavjee laid out a research agenda to improve this strategy, including the development of faster point-of-care (POC) tests, more effective vaccines for different indications, and immunomodulators to complement the antibiotics arsenal. He entreated the TB community to build more than just a TB program and aim for a community-based platform for better overall health care delivery. Keshavjee ended by showing how being able to diagnose and treat diseases is not only good for TB and a number of other infectious and noninfectious diseases but is also an important frame for biosecurity, as we have seen recently with COVID-19.

CHALLENGES AND INNOVATIONS

Presented by Eric Rubin, New England Journal of Medicine

Innovations and Translatable Lessons for TB Control from the COVID-19 Pandemic

Rubin highlighted innovations and translatable lessons from the COVID-19 pandemic that are applicable to diagnostics, therapeutics, and vaccines for TB.

Diagnostics

A major advance in diagnostics has been the scale-up and widespread implementation of polymerase chain reaction (PCR)-based testing during the COVID-19 pandemic, which holds promise for the application of similar technologies to pulmonary TB and perhaps other TB syndromes. Other innovative new technologies have been developed, such as rapid, cheap, POC diagnostics (Joung et al., 2020). However, implementation rates have been low for new tools such as rapid antigen-based testing, for example, and a POC PCR test has yet to be developed.

Therapeutics

Rubin noted the relative lack of progress during the COVID-19 pandemic in the domain of therapeutics, which has been largely caused by the lengthy therapeutic development timeline and the small existing pipeline for coronaviruses. Although there has been some success in developing glucocorticoids and other anti-inflammatory agents—and some modestly effective antivirals—no truly new agents have been developed and there have been no dramatic successes. Of the more than 200 clinical trials listed for COVID-19 therapeutics at the time of the workshop, many of them had been withdrawn, had repetitive trial designs, or had small sample sizes unlikely to yield useful results. These issues underscore the importance of coordination and thoughtfulness in the clinical trials enterprise to avoid redundancy and improve efficiency, especially for expensive and lengthy trials conducted across multiple groups. In the context of TB therapeutics, Rubin highlighted the need to maintain the drug development pipeline—which is already more robust for TB than it is for coronaviruses—and to continue designing and conducting cost-efficient clinical trials in the face of limited funding.

Vaccines

Rubin commended the unprecedentedly swift advances in the vaccine domain seen during the COVID-19 pandemic, from the rapid development and deployment of vaccines to extensive real-world safety testing for vaccine delivery methods. These efforts were bolstered by large randomized controlled trials conducted quickly while maintaining high quality (Polack et al., 2020; Tait et al., 2019). He noted that the success and widespread use of new technologies, such as messenger RNA (mRNA) and adenovirus vector vaccines, have broadened opportunities to rapidly test new antigens with less dependence on expensive and scarce adjuvants. However, he noted that the global case incidence for TB tends to be lower than case incidence for COVID-19, as the latter is in the midst of global outbreak. This disparity in case numbers contributes to a smaller effect size and complicates the conduct of vaccine trials. Rubin added that the identification of biomarkers that correlate with protection remain a critical knowledge gap in both TB and COVID-19 research. Without biomarkers or new and persuasive models, there are few available tools to assist with accelerating progress for large phase 3 trials.

NEW TECHNOLOGIES AND REMAINING GAPS IN TUBERCULOSIS DIAGNOSTICS

Presented by Soumya Swaminathan, World Health Organization

Swaminathan presented on new technologies and remaining gaps in TB diagnostics. She predicted that one long-term effect of COVID-19 is a likely increase in unreported and untreated cases of TB and other diseases for years to come. Modeling estimates suggest that 1.4 million fewer people received TB care in 2020 compared to 2019, with a 21 percent relative shortfall in TB case notifications during that period—giving rise to the potential for 500,000 additional TB deaths as a result (WHO, 2021b). The effect on the pediatric TB population is likely to be even greater, given the challenges associated with TB diagnosis in children such as children's difficulty producing sputum, their higher rates of extrapulmonary forms and disseminated forms of TB, and the lack of non–symptom-based sensitive and specific diagnostic tests. However, Swaminathan also noted that many countries have already begun to revitalize their TB programs, in some cases through conducting joint TB and COVID-19 response activities.

Innovations in Sample Types and Collection Methods

Swaminathan described a range of innovations in sample types and collection methods for POC or self-administered tests that have been developed for COVID-19 and could potentially be used for TB (Ruhwald et al., 2021). These include improvements in polyester swabs and new sampling protocols that use mouthwashes, oral swabs, or absorbent strips in facemasks. The use of easy-to-obtain samples, such as saliva, could transform TB and COVID-19 diagnosis by improving access to decentralized testing with drive-through facilities, mobile testing sites, community health workers, pharmacies, schools, and workplaces. Pharmacy-available, single-use self-testing kits also hold promise as rapid diagnostic tools, she added.

Innovations in Point-of-Care and Molecular Diagnostics

In the realm of POC diagnostics, Swaminathan highlighted several biomarker-based tests that use emerging technologies and that are currently under clinical evaluation and review, including the second-generation lateral flow lipoarabinomannan assay using urine samples. These tests have performed promisingly for people living with HIV/AIDS and may have potential to be expanded as a POC test for all forms of pulmonary TB. WHO plans to convene a Guideline Development Group in 2022 to review the clinical evidence for these tests (WHO, 2020). Swaminathan added that many countries have now scaled up their capacities to run molecular tests by using the foundations of existing TB and HIV programs, which had already centralized multidisease molecular platforms (e.g., HIV viral load assays) and could be further expanded to meet greater demand (Venkatesan, 2020). Several countries have used automated, cartridge-based molecular technologies, such as GeneXpert and TrueNAT, for both TB and COVID-19. However, such multidisease diagnostic platforms could be more robust, used more broadly in family health centers, and expanded in multiplex capabilities in order to achieve better cost and efficiency, said Swaminathan. She also noted that the broader use of molecular technologies and bidirectional testing would benefit TB diagnosis and reduce the reliance on suboptimal tools, such as smear microscopy (MacLean et al., 2020). It will not be possible to achieve TB elimination goals without more robust diagnostic tests, she warned.

Innovation in Digital Tools and Artificial Intelligence

Swaminathan remarked that the development of digital tools and AI have also accelerated during the COVID-19 pandemic (Budd et al., 2020). For example, digital solutions deployed for the mass dissemination of COVID-19 information such as smartphone apps and chat bots for education, risk communication, referrals, and contact tracing could be repurposed for TB to promote patient-centered care. Innovations in the application of AI to COVID-19 diagnostics, such as cough analyzers, digital stethoscopes, and automated X-ray interpretation—which had already been used for TB but saw expanded use during the pandemic—could be used for high-throughput screening and integrated testing for both TB and COVID-19, particularly if combined with portable X-ray units.

Innovations in Genomic Sequencing and Data Sharing

The capacity to rapidly collect and analyze large volumes of genomic sequencing data that was expanded and used during the COVID-19 pandemic could augment efforts to combat TB, noted Swaminathan. She remarked that the COVID-19 pandemic occurred during the digital era with the availability of real-time data sharing, large platforms, and user AI application analysis that enable rapid updates of data visualizations to inform public communications and direct the public health response. However, "TB still remains an analog disease, unfortunately, relying on paper-based systems and annual summary reporting. We really have to move away from that paradigm," she urged.

The knowledge gap around the genetic sequence-based detection of drug resistance to antibiotics (other than rifampicin) is widening, cautioned

Swaminathan. To address this gap, WHO has an ongoing effort to collaborate with global partners and countries worldwide to maintain a catalog of more than 17,000 mutations coming from a database with 38,000 isolates, with data on both whole genome sequencing and phenotypic drug susceptibility testing for 13 anti-TB drugs from 40 countries (WHO, 2021a). WHO is also planning to convene a Guideline Development Group for next-generation sequencing for TB in 2022 (WHO, 2020). The advances in genetic sequencing seen during the COVID-19 pandemic could be a major boon to TB diagnostics, she added. For instance, coupling data from next-generation sequencing to drug resistance would allow for the most relevant mutations for each drug to be identified and for future molecular tests to provide updated susceptibility information at the time of diagnosis.

In comparison, researchers have amassed nearly 2.5 million whole genome sequences for SARS-CoV-2 in the 2 years since the onset of the COVID-19 pandemic. COVID-19 variants have engendered renewed interest and investment in enhancing sequencing capacities in many countries. Such investments in robust data systems and data integration will benefit control efforts for TB as well as many other diseases, she added. Swaminathan suggested that WHO should take a central role in convening stakeholders to design data-sharing platforms for TB and other diseases that are similar to the database for COVID-19, which currently contains data from more than 350,000 individual patients from more than 60 countries. However, the dynamic and collaborative nature of this multilateral data platform will need to be balanced by safeguarding the confidence and interests of researchers from the Global South, she said.

Summary of Innovations

Swaminathan categorized emerging innovations from the COVID-19 pandemic into three major new domains: POC biomarkers in rapid diagnostic tests, multidisease platforms, and next-generation whole genome sequencing. She framed these efforts as being part of pandemic planning, preparedness, and coverage, thus warranting a focus on developing multidisease, multiplatform technologies and databases with crosscutting coverage across diseases. She pointed to the Access to COVID-19 Tools Accelerator (ACT-A) as an example of the progress that can be accomplished when multilateral stakeholders come together with a singular focus on addressing a disease.[5] Swaminathan concluded by reiterating key challenges and opportunities in advancing TB diagnostics (see Box 2-2).

---

[5] To learn more about the ACT-A, visit https://www.who.int/initiatives/act-accelerator (accessed August 18, 2021).

> **BOX 2-2**
> **Challenges and Opportunities in Advancing**
> **Tuberculosis Diagnostics**
>
> 1. Without new and more effective diagnostic tools, it is doubtful that global TB elimination goals will be met; this is a neglected and underfunded research area.
> 2. Digital tools will play a key role in the future, but more research is needed to accurately measure their effects on health outcomes.
> 3. Data sharing poses an important opportunity, but effective governance may be needed to ensure trust, confidentiality, and responsible use.
> 4. The three major domains that have seen advances during the COVID-19 pandemic are:
>   a. Point-of-care biomarker and other rapid diagnostic tests,
>   b. Multidisease platform diagnostics, and
>   c. Next-generation genetic sequencing.
> 5. Global multilateral mechanisms similar to the Access to COVID Tools Accelerator may serve as a model for developing and ensuring equitable access to address TB needs.
>
> SOURCE: Presented by Soumya Swaminathan on July 22, 2021.

IMPROVING TREATMENT REGIMENS AND VACCINE DEVELOPMENT

Presented by Emilio Emini, Bill & Melinda Gates Foundation

Emini explored challenges and opportunities related to developing and improving TB therapeutics and vaccines. He cautioned that TB would return to being the largest cause of infectious disease mortality worldwide after the COVID-19 pandemic is brought under control. The response to COVID-19 has illustrated the value of political commitment, global coordination, and robust funding in addressing infectious disease challenges. Although TB is difficult to address in many respects, Emini noted that the technical and scientific infrastructure for improved and effective versions of TB therapies and vaccines already exist. However, they must continue into the later phases of development, which will require—at minimum—the same level of global engagement and funding that supported the COVID-19 response.

Therapeutic Regimens

Emini explained that the rationale for developing new therapeutic regimens is to help reduce two gaps in the TB care cascade: the gap between diagnosis and treatment initiation, and the gap between treatment regimen completion and nonrelapsing cure. The current standard of care for TB treatment is too lengthy (i.e., 6 months, which contributes to loss to follow-up) and too toxic (associated with hepatitis, neuropathy, eye toxicity, skin reaction, and joint pain). It also has too many drug interactions, chief among them being with hormonal contraceptives and antiretroviral agents used to treat people living with HIV, who are particularly at risk of developing and dying from active TB. Consequently, the number of cured cases of DS TB has remained relatively stagnant over the past 5 years (WHO, 2020). During the same period, greater progress has been achieved in treating DR TB and MDR TB; this is attributable to rapid developments in the treatment for MDR TB, but these drug regimens are still too long and too toxic, he added.

Optimal Target Regimen Profile

Emini presented the optimal target regimen profile developed by BMGF to guide the development of new therapeutic regimens for TB. The criteria include:

1. Project to Accelerate New Treatments for Tuberculosis (Pan-TB): no requirement for drug sensitivity testing, ideally fewer patients lost to follow-up after diagnosis
2. Short: 3 months or less to achieve nonrelapsing cure, allowing for improved adherence, improved outcomes, and reduced transmission
3. Safe: minimal side effects to eliminate the need for baseline or ongoing safety monitoring and improve adherence
4. Simple: fully oral instead of injectable regimens, daily administration without drug–drug interactions to manage
5. Efficacy: noninferior to standard of care, minimizing gap between efficacy and effectiveness
6. Affordable: reducing financial barriers to uptake

Emini acknowledged that although this optimal target regimen profile is aspirational, some notable strides have been made toward achieving it. Several studies have already investigated whether various novel combinations of existing TB drugs could be noninferior to the current standard 6-month regimen in terms of treatment success over a shorter duration of time. Notably, the Tuberculosis Trials Consortium Study 31/AIDS Clinical Trials Group A5349[6] (TBTC Study 31/A5349) recently demonstrated noninferiority in

---

[6] For more information on Tuberculosis Trials Consortium Study 31/AIDS Clinical Trials Group A5349, see https://clinicaltrials.gov/ct2/show/NCT02410772 (accessed December 15, 2021).

treating DS TB using combinations of isoniazid, rifapentine, moxifloxacin, and pyrazinamide over a 4-month course.[7] This study demonstrates that shorter treatment regimens are achievable with the appropriate selection of drugs. However, Emini noted that the challenge going forward is determining which novel drugs or combination of drugs under development will fulfill other criteria of the optimal target regimen profile—particularly tolerability and ease of use—without requiring continuous clinical and drug monitoring.

Global Pipeline for New Tuberculosis Drugs

Emini noted that the Stop TB Partnership's Working Group on New TB Drugs has been tracking the global pipeline for new tuberculosis drugs,[8] which is extensive as of 2021, even without including the large number of drugs in the discovery phase. Many of these new drugs have emerged from large research collaborations between academic institutions and biopharmaceutical companies, such as the TB Drug Accelerator, the European Regimen Accelerator for Tuberculosis (ERA4TB) collaborative from the Innovative Medicines Initiative, and the recently established Project to Accelerate New Treatments for TB (PAN-TB) collaboration.[9,10] For example, the PAN-TB collaboration is bringing novel and potentially promising combinations of TB drugs into phase 2b clinical studies to assess and prioritize these candidates based on the optimal target regimen profile. However, a challenge on the horizon for these efforts will be garnering funding for the exponentially higher cost of large, extensive phase 3 trials needed to yield meaningful and actionable outcomes, he noted.

Vaccines

New vaccines are required to accelerate progress toward eliminating TB, said Emini. He noted that WHO's long-standing priority targets for TB vaccines include (1) preventing TB disease or infection in children and adults through vaccines that protect from TB by preventing infection or development of active disease, (2) preventing disease in neonates and infants through vaccines with a safety and efficacy profile comparable with Bacillus Calmette-Guérin (BCG) that protect against all forms of TB, and (3) protec-

---

[7] This is a recently completed clinical trial led by the Tuberculosis Trials Consortium at the U.S. CDC, with collaboration from the AIDS Clinical Trials Group funded by the National Institute of Allergy and Infectious Diseases. See CDC, 2020, and https://clinicaltrials.gov/ct2/show/NCT02410772 (accessed August 18, 2021).
[8] See https://www.newtbdrugs.org/pipeline/clinical (accessed August 18, 2021).
[9] For the TB Drug Accelerator Program from Global Health Progress, see https://globalhealthprogress.org/collaboration/tb-drug-accelerator-program (accessed August 18, 2021).
[10] For the IMI European Regimen Accelerator for Tuberculosis, see https://www.imi.europa.eu/projects-results/project-factsheets/era4tb (accessed August 18, 2021).

tion against TB recurrence following initial cure through therapeutic use of vaccines. Emini noted the particular lack of progress toward the second priority—developing a safe and efficacious vaccine for neonates and infants—and remarked that after a century of work in this area, BCG remains the only approved TB vaccine. There are currently a number of candidate TB vaccines in the global clinical pipeline, including some using an mRNA platform, that are in preclinical development and at various stages of clinical trials. Like the development of new treatment regimens, however, TB vaccine development also requires significant sources of funding for large and expensive phase 3 trials. Emini emphasized the significant funding challenges associated with advancing any vaccine candidate into a 20,000-participant phase 3 study: the chemistry, manufacturing, and control process development for the vaccine; epidemiology and capacity studies to identify critical trial sites with a high incidence of TB; and capacity building to support the study.

Emini highlighted two promising vaccine study candidates: BCG revaccination and the M72/AS01$_E$ vaccine. The potential efficacy of BCG revaccination was discovered unexpectedly when a statistically significant 50 percent decline in a signal for TB infection was observed in a control group that had essentially received a BCG revaccination during an unrelated study in 2018.[11] A second, larger study was initiated to determine if these results could be replicated,[12] which could lead to a major policy change for BCG use, he noted. M72/AS01$_E$ is a subunit vaccine that consists of M72—a fusion protein of two potential immunological targets from the pathogen—and the proprietary adjuvant AS01$_E$.[13] He noted that phase 2 trial results demonstrated an efficacy of only about 50 percent, but that level of efficacy could still have a substantial effect on TB epidemiology, particularly in high-burden settings.[14]

COLLECTIVE SOCIAL VALUE OF INFECTIOUS DISEASE INTERVENTIONS

Presented by Kevin Outterson, Boston University School of Law and CARB-X

Outterson explored the collective social value of infectious disease interventions. He discussed policy and economic considerations for building new

---

[11] For more information on the BCG revaccination study, see https://clinicaltrials.gov/ct2/show/NCT04152161 (accessed August 18, 2021).

[12] This study was still in progress at the time of the workshop.

[13] AS01$_E$ is approved for use as part of the Shingrix vaccine. For more information on the M72 vaccine trial, see Tait et al., 2019.

[14] There are conflicting views associated with revaccination. For additional perspectives, see Ahmed et al., 2021.

antibiotic development business models and identified potential translatable lessons for ongoing TB efforts.

Many organizations, funding streams, government agencies, and scientific communities associated with infectious diseases are separated by strong disciplinary boundaries drawn around diseases of focus. As a consequence, the disparate funding streams for efforts around antimicrobial resistance, TB, HIV, and other areas "becomes something of a zero-sum game in which we compete," he said. However, these groups could derive mutual benefit by learning from and sharing common experiences among each other, he added.

Broadening the Definition of Value for the Cooperative Production of Public Goods

It can be challenging for models for the cooperative production of public goods—such as treatments and interventions for infectious disease outbreak preparedness and response—to adopt a strategic perspective, noted Outterson. To address this issue, he suggested an alternative approach of adopting a broader view in defining the value of these antimicrobial interventions. For example, CARB-X encourages the framing of antibiotics as a "safety net" that enables modern medicine and creates a favorable risk–benefit calculus for common medical procedures such as cesarean sections and knee replacements, and cancer treatments. As with anti-TB interventions, it is difficult to quantify the value of effective antibiotics in an individual patient even though, as reported in a forthcoming study, infection is the second leading cause of death for people with cancer.

To elucidate the challenge of funding antimicrobial interventions, Outterson outlined five benefits gleaned from the health economics literature about the population-level benefits of effective antimicrobial therapy:

1. Spectrum—using narrow-spectrum antibiotics to reduce collateral damage to the microbiome, and broad-spectrum antibiotics to allow for interventions even when the diagnosis is not complete
2. Transmission—avoiding pathogen spread by treating patients effectively
3. Enablement—making other medical interventions possible (e.g., surgery)
4. Diversity—using a range of treatment options to reduce drug-resistance selection pressures
5. Insurance—having a backup in the event of a new, sudden, or significant increase in drug resistance

From a funding perspective, each of these benefits is associated with billions or even trillions of dollars' worth of population- or social-level value, and it is difficult for the current market to reimburse the researchers for those forms of value, said Outterson. In the antimicrobial space, the result is that traditional market pricing mechanisms do not appropriately incentivize novel antimicrobial development, thus undermining the entire sector. For example, 7 of 18 new antimicrobials approved by the U.S. Food and Drug Administration (FDA) since 2010 have been either associated with bankruptcy or withdrawn from marketing applications in Europe, generally owing to the pharmaceutical companies' position that the forecasted profit margins in Europe do not justify the costs of a second market authorization. To provide context with the sales of other pharmaceutical products, Outterson shared that the annual U.S. sales for all branded antibacterials approved by FDA since 2010 total around $720 million in the United States, which is less than the U.S. annual revenue generated by the most profitable single oncology drug.[15]

Building New Therapeutic Development Business Models to Catalyze Development

In the face of this economic problem, the antimicrobial industry has been considering changing its business models in ways that could potentially benefit the TB community, said Outterson. Major funding organizations typically support either basic research coupled with early discovery or late-stage clinical development; CARB-X has tried to bridge that binary divide. He acknowledged that the TB drug development effort has the advantages of more coordinated pipelines and strategically set target product profiles to guide development, but there is an opportunity to work collaboratively across funding and research silos and reward the development of antimicrobials—including TB drugs—based on their social value. He suggested making such an argument by encouraging resource allocation based on clinical baseline needs and strategic planning between outbreaks, rather than allocating resources during emergencies to combat microbial threats when they arise. Rather than competing for funding streams, experts from different disciplines of microbial threats could be encouraged to discuss their common needs and the broader social values of innovation.

Outterson also suggested that governments could finance antimicrobial innovation through a "subscription" business model, whereby an established amount of government funding is steadily available to drug developers regardless of the actual market demand for new antibiotics. In addition to increasing financial incentives for companies, this would help to maintain a robust research, development, and manufacturing ecosystem capable of supporting supply chain redundancies and remaining resilient to perturbations in market demand.

---

[15] The recently published article found sales to be $714.3 million in the U.S. for branded, on-patent antibacterials. See Outterson et al. (2022).

Outterson concluded by connecting the new Advanced Research Projects Agency for Health (ARPA-H) to his call for collaboration, suggesting that it could serve as a platform for sharing practical experiences—for example, regarding how to operate at scale effectively or prioritize candidates within a pipeline. He noted that ARPA-H is likely to receive roughly $3 billion dollars in appropriations from Congress to fund health product development through a model similar to the Defense Advanced Research Projects Agency's model for funding technical and engineering innovation. He noted that efforts to break down silos between infectious disease disciplines will help to capitalize on future opportunities.

DISCUSSION

Considerations in Improving Diagnostic Capacities

Castro asked about the feasibility and potential level of support from WHO and the global community for replacing rapid PCR test kits for COVID-19 with a multiplexed version capable of testing for both COVID-19 and TB. This approach could enable widespread screening of patients with respiratory symptoms, while potentially helping to recover funding and renew case-finding efforts in TB-endemic areas, he suggested. Rubin replied that it might be possible to repurpose the COVID-19 rapid tests to include TB, but it would require dealing with technical issues related to specimen preparation for TB testing. Specifically, it would be challenging to reconcile sample processing for the two diseases in the same test kit, given that the current standard diagnostic specimen type is sputum for TB and nasal swab or saliva sample for COVID-19. Castro then asked about the status of commercializing a nonsputum POC test for TB. Emini said that it may be feasible to couple PCR testing for COVID-19 and TB using oral samples—bypassing the sputum-processing issue—but further major challenges would arise in breaching the organisms' structures to access their genomes because the causative agents for TB and COVID-19 are very different. He noted that the evidence base and diagnostic algorithms for detecting the presence of bacteria or volatile biomarkers in exhaled breath samples are under development, but those tests are not yet close to clinical application.

Keshavjee responded to a comment about the 2012 buy-down agreement, which was intended to improve countries' access to the tests and spur market demand. However, it unintentionally decoupled price determination from production volume,[16] which required negotiating the price of the new

---

[16] For an analysis of the buy-down, see Branigan (2020).

GeneXpert cartridges down to $5 per test.[17] Keshavjee explained that this resulted in limited uptake of the GeneXpert test, which precluded widespread community screening and heightened the reliance on smear microscopy for diagnosing TB, though it has lower sensitivity (WHO, 2011). Community screening conducted through AI-aided X-ray screening, which would cost less than $1 per person, followed by a confirmatory genetic test (e.g., GeneXpert, TrueNAT) could be a more diagnostically accurate and cost-effective strategy, he added. An economically priced diagnostic test would make the expansion of large-scale community diagnostic testing capacity feasible.

Economic Considerations and Implications for Program Design

Rubin asked whether price is generally a driving factor in front-end development or a later consideration once a product reaches market. Emini replied that although price is often considered up front, it is affected by multiple variables—chiefly, volume and competition. He offered the example of a buy-down, in which negotiation can modulate the volume of goods, but in the absence of competition, a single supplier would still control the price. The BMGF led a buy-down initiative for HIV self-testing in a number of African countries, where a system was built to introduce competition into the market. Consequently, the initial buy-down helped to lower product prices early on and to generate data showing the effect of HIV self-testing, while competition between multiple suppliers kept prices low over time.

While price-control systems hold promise, a concern is that prices for new TB drug combination regimens may not be able to compete with the low cost of the classic combination treatment of isoniazid, rifampicin, and pyrazinamide, Emini cautioned. He reiterated that a major challenge in improving TB treatment outcomes is finding a way to balance the price that the market will bear with the cost that society is asked to bear, which is an important prospective consideration for program and intervention development. Key questions include how the drugs will be used, who will pay for them, and what balance is optimal from both the societal and market perspectives, he added.

Outterson acknowledged Emini's distinction between cost of goods and price, adding that the introduction of social value as a consideration further distinguishes that difference and, moreover, can shift a company's focus from deriving revenue from market mechanisms to other reimbursements for its activities, including research and development (R&D). This concept, known

---

[17] Organizations involved in negotiating the 2012 buy-down agreement included the BMGF, the U.S. President's Emergency Plan for AIDS Relief, the U.S. Agency for International Development, and Unitaid; see http://www.stoptb.org/wg/new_diagnostics/assets/documents/News_XpertPrice_21Aug12.pdf (accessed August 18, 2021).

as "delinkage," is exemplified by the subscription-style funding model of the PASTEUR Act, which delinks a company's reward from sales volume, unit sales, and unit price. Outterson pointed out that delinkage is not a market mechanism; instead, it recognizes that "the market doesn't function to deliver social value when you're doing it through individual transactions on individual patients, so it's the difference between patient-level and population-level reimbursement." He added that the interventions discussed at the workshop could be made broadly available at little to no cost to the public if there were a way to appropriately reward companies.

Outterson added that the ultimate cost of goods is a consideration early on in the preclinical development life cycle at CARB-X; the optimizations for cost structure and adaptive research into product characteristics (e.g., stability, shelf life) are initiated closer to clinical trials. This type of optimization work receives special funding from the UK government. In circumstances of limited competition—such as the period of market exclusivity for patent-protected drugs—CARB-X has had success in contractually mandating global stewardship and access principles at the start of funding, he added.[18]

Bridging Silos and Shifting Paradigms

Rubin observed that the TB control community appears divided into two camps: one focused on developing new tools and interventions, the other on implementing them. He noted that the path from development to implementation is not always fluid, pointing out that CARB-X and the BMGF have tried to approach this translational medicine challenge by envisioning the target characteristics and usability of the end product early on. Rubin also pointed out that while breakthroughs and innovations could transform current programs, many underused interventions and tools for TB elimination are available right now. He called for movement forward in both areas by improving the implementation of existing tools while also working to develop better tools for the future.

Paradigm Shift to Improve Implementation of Existing Tools

Keshavjee remarked upon opportunities to create large effects with small changes to current TB programs. To illustrate, he suggested the policy changes of (1) shifting to community-level screening combined with commitments to contact tracing for prophylaxis and (2) establishing a mechanism for coordinated, rapid clinical trial studies, similar to some of the efforts made during the COVID-19 pandemic.

---

[18] Outterson noted that this is a concept that CARB-X adapted from their funders, including the BMGF and the Wellcome Trust.

Castro inquired about institutional changes or implementation arrangements needed to effectively support the search-treat-prevent strategy. Keshavjee suggested that TB control programs could reconfigure their principles and operations to frame TB as a social disease, rather than a disease of individuals.

This reconfiguration could lead TB control programs to extend beyond providing DOTS therapy for positive cases to creating household screening systems, he said. Although the household screening model would require more staffing, testing resources, and medications, especially in resource-limited settings, Keshavjee maintained that this would facilitate a step toward expanding TB control programs into general health care delivery platforms equipped to address other common diseases (e.g., diabetes, hypertension). An additional benefit of this type of robust, on-the-ground health care system would be immediate increased capacity for uptake and deployment of new treatments, vaccines, or diagnostic tests. This could also contribute to fostering innovations by providing rollout assurances and market access, he added.

Castro asked if studies of human–systems interactions might be incorporated alongside platform development to improve the end-user experience, reduce waste, and improve efficiency and effectiveness. Keshavjee responded that any treatment model has a behavioral economics component. For example, the conditional cash transfers described by Kim have a twofold benefit: stimulating local economies and encouraging participation in public health efforts to eliminate disease. He acknowledged that these methods have not been used widely in controlling TB, but they represent an opportunity for programmatic improvement by taking community contexts into account. He suggested that each TB program should be asking, "How do you actually interact with [people] and the community in a way that people will want to get screened, and people will want to take treatments?"

Paradigm Shift to Articulate the Biosecurity and Social Values of Tuberculosis Elimination

Keshavjee made the case that the lack of community health care delivery capacity for diagnosis, screening, and treatment constitutes a biosecurity emergency. To address this issue, he suggested calling for funding agencies to support comprehensive health programs rather than tying their funding to specific diseases or activities. Related workshops and organizations might have a role in conveying this need to stakeholders. Keshavjee cited evidence from a colleague's forthcoming study, which estimated that each missed (i.e., untreated) TB patient in India—assuming each person infects an additional 1.5 people annually over 5 years—costs the national economy $6,000. Cassell noted that such economic data can bolster compelling policy arguments for TB control.

Monique Mansoura, executive director of global health security and biotechnology at the MITRE Corporation, reflected on the cost of inaction for TB and potential competing health care needs in a community. She asked about the evidence base on the cost-effectiveness and synergistic outcomes associated with addressing TB and another prevalent disease (e.g., diabetes). Keshavjee shared two examples from TB programs that are also screening for diabetes and hypertension: the Resource Group for Advocacy and Community Health (REACH) in India and Advance Access & Delivery in Durban, South Africa.[19,20] Both programs have detected high rates of diabetes among people testing positive for TB in addition to significant rates of hypertension. Both conditions are generally easy and affordable to treat compared to TB, he noted, so it is relatively manageable for TB control field teams to take on treatment services for diabetes and hypertension in addition to their TB-related work. Keshavjee was hopeful that in the future, these programs would operate from unified funding streams, supply chains, and equipment for the treatment of many other health conditions that are currently disconnected.

Castro asked how to balance the competing needs for vertical programs and disease-specific objectives with broad, integrated health systems. He added that instead of viewing silos as structures to be dismantled, he sees them as centers of excellence that need to be connected. Outterson framed the social value of eliminating disease threats as the basis for integrated health systems and a bridge connecting different silos of expertise. For instance, the social value of elimination could be used to inform prioritization and balance objectives in funding decisions. He contrasted the rapid successes of the response to COVID-19, in which a large amount of capital was spent in a short period of time on a focused objective—possible, in part, because of the broadly perceived high value of elimination—with a hypothetical scenario in which that same level of effort and funding were spread out over a 20-year period. The latter case would be seen as a failure, but is actually similar to the approach taken for many other infectious diseases including TB. Outterson proposed that this type of health system strengthening could be thought of as broad-spectrum defenses against unknown or unknowable microbial threats. He remarked,

> The preparedness value of that is immense, and it crosses all silos[;] because it's not a preparedness system to surveil for any of our particular diseases, it should be something that surveils for all infectious diseases, and...even chronic diseases that aren't infectious.

---

[19] More information about the REACH TB Network is available from https://www.reachtbnetwork.org (accessed December 15, 2021).

[20] More information about Advance Access & Delivery is available from http://www.advanceaccessanddelivery.org (accessed December 15, 2021).

Closing Remarks

In closing, Cassell entreated the audience and participants to work toward developing the goals laid out by Kim in the opening presentation. To illustrate the urgency of addressing TB, she offered the statistic that roughly 500,000 people fall ill with MDR TB every year, yet that number has not changed since the very first WHO report on MDR TB more than 20 years ago. In addition, this statistic is difficult to interpret given that the actual burden of TB was likely higher than reported. A previous workshop proceedings from the Institute of Medicine states that only one half of one percent of patients diagnosed with MDR TB were being treated (IOM, 2012). Given that TB is spread via aerosol, the actual number of MDR TB cases in 2022 is likely significantly higher. Cassell emphasized that determining the social value of ending TB is an important task that may require innovative economic research and policy making to be achieved.

3

Detection

The first session of the second part of the workshop centered on the state of tuberculosis (TB) detection worldwide and advances that are currently underway to improve case finding, diagnostics, and case notification. The session began with progress updates on efforts to build a TB-free world by Jennifer Adams, acting assistant administrator, Bureau for Global Health at the U.S. Agency for International Development (USAID); Eric Goosby, professor of medicine at University of California, San Francisco, director of the Center for Global Health Delivery, Diplomacy and Economics at the Institute for Global Health Sciences, and United Nations (UN) Special Envoy on Tuberculosis; and Matteo Zignol, head of the Prevention, Care, and Innovation Unit of the Global TB Programme at the World Health Organization (WHO).

Matthew McMahon, director of the Small Business Education and Entrepreneurial Development Office at the National Institutes of Health, then discussed efforts to rapidly accelerate the development of diagnostics technology for COVID-19 and highlighted lessons learned that could potentially be applied to TB diagnostics. Next was a panel discussion on diagnostic advances that featured four panelists. Morten Ruhwald, head of tuberculosis at the Foundation for Innovative New Diagnostics, discussed point-of-care molecular platforms for diagnosis of TB and other infectious respiratory diseases. Zvi Marom, chief executive officer and founder at BATM Advanced Communications, described his organization's innovative approach to tackling TB amid the COVID-19 pandemic by focusing on substantially reducing the cost of diagnostic testing and to initiate TB treatment rapidly after an accurate diagnosis. Luan Vo, chief executive officer at Friends for International Tuberculosis Relief, presented on the implementation of ultraportable X-ray technology and the use of AI for X-ray interpretation for TB detection in Vietnam. Kaiser Shen, senior TB diagnostic technical advisor at USAID's Sustaining Technical and Analytic Resources project, shared insights from his work at USAID on point-of-care (POC) TB diagnostics, TB diagnostic networks, and implementation challenges.

The session then shifted focus to highlight efforts to improve adherence, infection control capacities, and cost-effectiveness. Amir Khan, executive director at Interactive Research and Development (IRD), discussed the comprehensive approach to COVID-19 and TB testing implemented in Pakistan by adapting IRD's model of integrated community response to TB control. Bruce Thomas, founder and managing director of the Arcady Group, described how digital adherence technologies (DATs) can facilitate differentiated and virtual care for persons affected by TB. Monique Mansoura, executive director for Global Health and Biotechnology at the MITRE Corporation, explored innovative strategies to synergize investments in health care systems with a focus on whether cancer and TB care can protect against pandemics. Edward Nardell, professor of medicine at Harvard Medical School and the Harvard T.H. Chan School of Public Health and physician at Brigham and Women's Hospital, outlined environmental transmission control lessons that can be gleaned from efforts to control TB over many decades and efforts to control COVID-19 since 2020. Gavin Churchyard, founder and chief executive officer of the Aurum Institute, discussed gaps and opportunities in the management of latent TB infection and barriers to the implementation of tuberculosis preventive therapy (TPT). The session was moderated by Lucica Ditiu, executive director of the Stop TB Partnership.

USAID'S COMMITMENT TO ADDRESSING TUBERCULOSIS WORLDWIDE

Presented by Jennifer Adams, United States Agency for International Development

Adams described how USAID has made a long-standing commitment to work with partners in addressing TB worldwide by reaching every person with TB, curing people in need of treatment, preventing new infections, and stopping the progression of TB from infection to active disease. Strong gains have been made over the past two decades. Between 2000 and 2019, more than 60 million lives were saved globally, TB incidence decreased by 29 percent, TB mortality decreased by 47 percent, and TB case notifications increased by 126 percent, Adams noted. USAID has contributed a focus on research and clinical trials to this effort, including the introduction and scaling up of new drugs and shorter treatment regimens and the development of stronger diagnostic tools and networks. In 2018, TB garnered renewed energy and attention with the UN High-Level Meeting on Ending TB, which set ambitious targets and generated increases in domestic resources and political commitments.

The COVID-19 pandemic has had devastating effects on the global TB response—in addition to other public health issues—and continues to dim the prospects of meeting the ambitious UN targets, said Adams. The social, economic, and biomedical consequences of the pandemic have created a perfect storm for TB and other public health issues. She noted that the COVID-19 pandemic has been particularly devastating for the poorest and most vulnerable populations in low- and middle-income countries (LMICs). These populations are more likely to suffer from other health problems, including malnutrition, and they often live in overcrowded spaces that increase their risk of contracting COVID-19 and TB. Adams recounted the waves of COVID-19 she witnessed while serving as the USAID mission director in Mozambique, the first of which caused all clinics to close, thereby interrupting access to TB care and other health services. Reports from Mozambique's national TB program indicated that the number of people diagnosed with TB dropped by almost half during the pandemic. Simultaneously, TB personnel and services were repurposed and deployed in the response to COVID-19. Their experience in case detection, contact tracing, and airborne infection control were essential for the new and unprecedented pandemic, said Adams. She remarked that the focus should now be on ending the long-term negative effects that COVID-19 is having on other health needs, particularly on TB and in countries with very high TB burdens. This involves renewing commitments, reinvesting in infrastructure to meet unmet needs, and contributing to a consensus on how to best prepare for future pandemics. Much of what is being discussed in terms of pandemic preparedness and response directly aligns with TB interventions.

The COVID-19 pandemic has led to alarming drops in the number of people tested and treated for TB, Adams remarked. USAID focuses on TB programming in 23 countries, and reports indicate that 1 million fewer people had access to TB diagnosis and treatment in 2020 as compared to 2019, representing over a 20 percent decline. Partnerships between national TB programs and the Global Fund to Fight AIDS, Tuberculosis and Malaria are needed to mitigate this decline, and USAID has developed a 9-month recovery effort in seven countries with high TB burdens that have been most affected by pandemic-related service disruptions. These recovery activities focus on increasing access to services—including simultaneous testing for TB and COVID-19—with the aim of strengthening diagnostic networks, launching awareness campaigns, conducting community-based case finding, and expanding the use and availability of adherence tools. Adams noted that new tools and technologies, some of which were rapidly developed and adopted to support services during the COVID-19 pandemic, will be critical in helping countries to recover and restore public health efforts. Examples of innovation supported within USAID include computerized pillboxes, screening and tracking mobile applications, and video adherence monitoring technology.

The scale-up of all-oral treatment regimens has been critical in continuing multidrug-resistant (MDR) TB treatment for patients throughout the restrictions and lockdowns brought on by the pandemic, Adams remarked. Combinations of new regimes and technologies should continue beyond the COVID-19 pandemic, and USAID is focusing on mitigating the long-term consequences of COVID-19 on TB with interventions that are most effective. Adams noted that the use of TB systems and staff to combat COVID-19 reflects the value of TB investments. The investments made thus far by USAID and others have effectively built systems within communities that include primary and even tertiary care to cure people and save lives. Addressing TB in current times will require increased investment and political commitment, as well as innovation, adaptation, and aggressive action toward global targets to end TB.

BUILDING A TUBERCULOSIS-FREE WORLD: PROGRESS UPDATE

Presented by Eric Goosby, University of California, San Francisco

Goosby provided a progress update on efforts to build a TB-free world. He remarked that despite being preventable and curable, TB remains the largest infectious disease killer worldwide, while the burden of MDR TB continues to spread. Although effective diagnostics and therapeutics are available, their implementation has been hampered by the lack of sustained political commitment. TB control programs need to continuously outpace the transmission of mycobacteria through the population, yet governmental support of such efforts has been inconsistent over time. Further complicating the situation, the COVID-19 pandemic has displaced TB response efforts that will need to be reestablished and repositioned, he added.

Recent Milestones in Tuberculosis Control Advocacy

Before stepping down from the office of UN Secretary-General, Ban Ki-moon called for action to reinvigorate a global response to end the TB epidemic. Critical groundwork for addressing endemic diseases has been laid by efforts focused on human immunodeficiency virus (HIV), including the President's Emergency Plan for AIDS Relief and the partnerships created between ministries of health in many countries with overlapping high burdens of HIV and TB. These collaborations gave reason to hope for rapid dialogue to facilitate a strengthened TB response and a more orchestrated universal health coverage agenda. Goosby described a coordinated effort between the Stop TB Partnership, the Global Fund, and the HIV community in lobbying for a high-level meeting on TB that served as an opportunity to identify priority-strengthening targets and encourage country-specific implementation efforts. Leading up to the meeting, working groups highlighted the need for legislative engagement in prioritizing TB when responding to ministry of health budgetary requests, said Goosby. Therefore, legislative leaders were targeted for education, and many of these leaders expressed surprise at the level of TB burden in their countries. Representatives from the Global TB Caucus attended G20 meetings to raise TB awareness for leaders from high-TB-burden countries. Stop TB focused advocacy efforts in Nigeria, India, and other countries to engage leaders in programming offered by their organization. Within that cohort of leaders, Stop TB worked to identify, create, and strengthen leadership to advocate for the prioritization and funding of TB response efforts among legislators.

Investment Priorities for Tuberculosis Control

In 2019, the Lancet Commission on Tuberculosis established five priority investment areas for addressing TB (Reid et al., 2019) (see Box 3-1), which recognized the importance of accounting for each country's met and unmet needs when developing implementation strategies for effective TB diagnostic and treatment efforts (Reid and Yamey, 2019). However, collaborative attempts to converge efforts by the UN, WHO, and the Stop TB Partnership have not yet gained traction, he remarked. Although conversations are taking place, they have yet to translate into budgetary expansion and programmatic implementation decisions that expand TB capability worldwide. Goosby added that G20 countries can take a leadership role and emphasize the need for G7 countries to continue to expand their participation and financial support.

To create an enabling environment and hold countries accountable for making progress to end TB—the fifth priority of the Lancet Commission—Goosby suggested (1) recognizing the powerful role to be played by TB survivors and advocates; (2) committing to address drivers of TB including HIV, undernutrition, and pollution; and (3) advancing the universal health coverage agenda, given the foundation it provides for the prevention and treatment of all health conditions. Certain diseases such as HIV and TB have received unique funding, but expansion of the entire health care delivery platform to the population would strengthen efforts focused on specific diseases, Goosby stated. Ministers of health can be their countries' strongest advocates for budgetary prioritization, but effective advocacy requires analyzing and understanding the situation and translating it into a narrative that attracts funding.

> **BOX 3-1**
> **Investment Priorities for Ending Tuberculosis**
>
> 1. Provide patient-centered services to all seeking tuberculosis care.
> 2. Reach high-risk people with screening and prevention programs.
> 3. Develop new diagnostics, therapies, and vaccines.
> 4. Invest funds necessary to end tuberculosis.
> 5. Hold countries and stakeholders accountable for making progress to end tuberculosis.
>
> SOURCES: Presented by Eric Goosby on September 14, 2021; Reid et al., 2019.

COVID-19 Pandemic: Consequences and Opportunities for Tuberculosis

In the United States, the COVID-19 pandemic has displaced the national focus from diseases such as HIV and TB, noted Goosby. Many of the experts in the HIV and TB communities have the skill sets needed to identify, understand, and contain a new virus moving into a population. As a result, the United States and many European countries drew talent and human resources from the TB/HIV arena, and built upon those existing systems of care, to mount their responses to the COVID-19 pandemic. Moreover, the pandemic accelerated progress through the stages of identification, diagnostic capability, discerning high-risk groups, and prioritizing high-risk groups for diagnosis, treatment, and eventually, vaccination.

Although the International Health Regulations (IHR) of 2005 established a consensus about the need to strengthen outbreak surveillance capacities, this has not yet been achieved—which is particularly striking in countries where a pandemic threat is more likely to emerge. Goosby suggested that the United States should exercise leadership in G7 discussions to bring the issue of surveillance to G20 and establish the expectation that an IHR surveillance system will be built, monitored, and maintained. He proposed that countries that cannot afford to build surveillance systems should be accommodated by having a system built for them, but they should assume and maintain the responsibility for implementing the system. Additionally, each country's system should be connected to the ministry of health, which should preserve the information system and use it to detect COVID-19 and other diseases. Goosby warned against creating parallel systems of surveillance, which has happened in the past with HIV.

Goosby added that the Biden administration has discussed strategies to increase pandemic preparedness by building upon established platforms, such as those for TB and HIV. These platforms would be strengthened and expanded to accommodate the demands from any new threat, such as COVID-19. Strengthening the capability for global response would also facilitate the identification and mitigation of inequities in capacities and distribution of resources. Questions persist as to where that capability will reside and which entities will be responsible for different components, he added, noting that dialogue around national security versus global health programming remains in equilibrium.

Discussion

Referencing a divide between the national security and global health communities, Mansoura asked how these communities can be brought together in recognizing the security elements and economic effects of TB. Goosby replied that the cultures within the national security and global health communities are quite different and are unfamiliar with one another. The national security community is viewed as being aligned with a military agenda that defines a threat as the topography of the area where it originated. The medical community tends to be uncomfortable with that perspective, and therein lies a tension, he remarked. Global health concerns can be overlaid on requests for resources for a governmental security expansion—requests that are unlikely to be denied—because global health issues can be justifiably aligned with funding that is motivated by security concerns, said Goosby. This process can be conducted in collaboration with, rather than controlled by, policy makers at the National Security Council.

Goosby voiced his confidence that this process will eventually take place, while acknowledging delays caused by disagreement around who should control the process and by a lack of sustained focus on the issue. He contended that rather than taking a solo approach to funding or implementing efforts, U.S. leadership can back a position that pivots global support into activities that expand capacity within each country. Such a path can incorporate needs related to the COVID-19 pandemic to create a sustainable system of agreements and synergies to address future pandemic threats. Goosby noted that the United States has the gravitas to convene discussions in the G7 and G20 summits around creating such a system. The current moment presents an opportunity to invigorate global health leadership. Rather than position itself as "the elephant in the room," the United States can bring a herd of elephants into the room, said Goosby.

Marcos Espinal, director of the Department of Communicable Diseases and Environmental Determinants of Health at the Pan American Health Organization, said that the United States, the G7 countries, and WHO are positioned to lead the development of a pandemic preparedness platform, and this will be the focus of a special session of the World Health Assembly in November 2021. In 2015, WHO initiated emergency response reforms following the Ebola epidemic the year prior, including the creation of the WHO Health Emergencies Programme. However, a lack of connectivity between various platforms has emerged during the COVID-19 pandemic, said Espinal. The United States has an opportunity to use well-developed platforms—such as those for TB and HIV—for expansion into pandemic preparedness. He noted that the COVID-19 pandemic has created massive disruptions for TB and HIV programs and the administration of TB, diphtheria-tetanus-pertussis, and polio vaccines in Latin America and the Caribbean. Thus, major gains in the international community are currently threatened by the current pandemic, and preparedness is needed before the next pandemic.

Goosby stated that the United States has an opportunity to lead the pandemic preparedness effort in a respectful way that enhances the global perspective of U.S. leadership. Such an approach would avoid creating "islands of excellence" that cause and perpetuate disparities between those that benefit from the bilateral infusion of resources for a single disease and those that do not. Instead, a continued resource commitment can be used to strengthen ministries of health and expand their platforms, because this is the most sustainable way to preserve services for the population, said Goosby. The fifth priority from the Lancet Commission on Tuberculosis is holding countries and stakeholders accountable for making progress toward ending TB (Reid et al., 2019). When nations implement programs in other countries, this fragments responsibility and dilutes the ability to sustain and increase the effect of investments. Instead, systems and services that clearly designate the countries in which they are implemented as responsible for maintenance and continued performance should be created, Goosby remarked. The demands of the COVID-19 pandemic present an opportunity to reevaluate the global health development portfolio and expand platforms implemented in partnership with leaders responsible for the target population. This approach incorporates an understanding of accountability that has been missing, Goosby stated. He added that the United States could adopt this approach to create sustainable programs instead of solutions that last for 3 to 5 years and then disappear.

Eltony Mugomeri, lecturer at Africa University (AU) and project manager of a TB partnership program with AU and Zimbabwe's Ministry of Health, remarked that countries with a high burden of TB need to strengthen information systems and diagnostic technologies—such as mobile X-ray machines and video conferencing equipment—while building capacity within a short time frame. He asked how affected countries can establish synergies to address these challenges. Goosby replied that the strongest approach is in-country civil society partners collaborating with the ministry of health to approach funders together. The current allocation of investments within the health care delivery system can be examined for repositioning opportunities. As new resources come in—for example, pandemic support—decision makers can examine their potential best uses in alignment with other needs within the same community. Additionally, a limited role for public–private partnerships should be circumscribed, suggested Goosby. Although public–private partnerships should not displace or dilute lines of responsibility, the private sector contains resources and expertise in procurement distribution systems, budget management, and human resource (HR) management that can benefit ministries of health. Shared HR positions, sites, and referral mechanisms can be formally defined to avoid duplicating systems of care that cross over from public to private, said Goosby.

REALITIES OF MULTIDRUG-RESISTANT TUBERCULOSIS

Presented by Matteo Zignol, World Health Organization

Zignol focused on the global burden and trends in MDR TB, the associated challenges that it poses to TB control, and progress in the treatment of MDR TB.

Burden and Trends in Multidrug-Resistant Tuberculosis

Zignol opened by presenting data about the global burden of TB and its epidemiological trends drawn from WHO's *2020 Global Tuberculosis Report* (WHO, 2020). In 2019, one-quarter of the world's population was infected with TB and an estimated 10 million people developed TB disease. About 815,000 of those 10 million individuals had HIV-associated TB and 465,000 had MDR TB or rifampicin-resistant (RR) TB. The same year, roughly 1.4 million people died of TB—including deaths attributed to HIV/TB—and 208,000 died of HIV-associated TB, while 182,000 people died of MDR/RR TB. The majority of individuals with MDR/RR TB are located in a small number of countries with emerging economies, including India, China, Russia, South Africa, Indonesia, and the Philippines. While TB is a disease of the poor, the majority of the TB burden, particularly for MDR/RR TB, is located in growing economies.

The discussion of drug-resistant (DR) TB is typically framed in terms of resistance to rifampicin, which is one of the most powerful first-line TB drugs. However, Zignol noted that the total global burden of DR TB—which also includes isoniazid-resistant/rifampicin-susceptible TB—far exceeds that of RR TB alone (WHO, 2020). The combined burden of isoniazid resistance or rifampicin resistance amounts to about 1.5 million persons with TB that is resistant to the two most powerful first-line drugs every year.

Trends in Levels of Tuberculosis Drug Resistance

Despite the development of advanced surveillance systems, TB surveillance is not yet adequate, said Zignol. In particular, the availability of TB data is limited in countries with high burdens of RR TB and, as of 2019, some countries had no data on RR TB. Further, many of the countries with data on RR TB have collected data on new case rates only a few times in the past 25 years, making it difficult to establish trends. Fortunately, data on MDR TB trends are available from multiple high-burden countries, including Azerbaijan, Belarus, Kazakhstan, Kyrgyzstan, Myanmar, Peru, Moldova, Russia, Tajikistan, Thailand, Ukraine, and Vietnam. In many of these countries, rates of both TB and MDR TB are declining, with MDR TB declining at a slower rate than TB in some settings. In other countries, such as the Russian Federation, TB is declining while MDR TB is not.

Zignol discussed findings from a 2017 study that modeled projected trends in the proportions of MDR TB and extensively drug-resistant (XDR) TB in India, the Philippines, Russia, and South Africa (Sharma et al., 2017). The study predicted that the proportion of MDR TB and XDR TB will increase in the next 20 years, with the expected increase in proportions of MDR TB and XDR TB linked to the expected decline in overall TB incidence. The reduction of TB incidence may foster the accumulation of drug resistance and create more favorable conditions for the transmission of DR TB, he added. A 2021 study projected the effect of a post-exposure vaccine on RR TB in India, Russia, China, and Nigeria, finding that post-exposure vaccines could have a favorable effect on RR TB incidence rates (Fu et al., 2021). Zignol added that post-exposure vaccines may also favorably affect the transmission of DR TB.

Challenges for Tuberculosis Control

Zignol discussed specific challenges for TB control posed by the COVID-19 pandemic in terms of diagnosis, notifications, and mortality. The COVID-19 pandemic had a substantial effect on TB notification rates. Global TB notifications dropped from 6.3 million in 2019 to 4.9 million in 2020, 28 percent less than the expected notifications for 2020. In some countries, the shortfall from expected notifications in 2020 was as high as 40 percent (WHO, 2021b). The COVID-19 pandemic is also expected to influence TB mortality in a manner correlated with shortfalls in case detection, leading to an estimated excess TB mortality of approximately 500,000 deaths.

Furthermore, the COVID-19 pandemic has reduced TB diagnosis rates, largely because of the limited availability of molecular tests for detecting TB and DR TB, said Zignol. Of the 10 million new people with TB disease every year, only 7.1 million are notified and 5.9 million of those are pulmonary

TB cases. Only 3.4 million of those receive a bacteriologically confirmed TB diagnosis, and only one out of five of those individuals are diagnosed with rapid tests, which are the most sensitive and specific available. Thus, only about 20 percent of people who develop TB disease each year actually receive the proper diagnosis, he said. However, RR TB testing coverage among bacteriologically confirmed TB cases is now increasing; nearly 60 percent of new cases and 80 percent of repeat cases received testing for rifampicin resistance in 2019. The testing coverage rate for fluoroquinolone resistance among RR TB cases was 71 percent in 2019. He added that the lack of a POC diagnostic test for TB is a pressing concern and low-hanging fruit for improving TB control. Such a test could be quickly developed and would substantially strengthen global TB control efforts.

Advances and Progress in Tuberculosis Treatment

Zignol highlighted recent advances and progress in TB treatment. More treatment regimens are available than ever before, with many new shorter regimens now available for both DS and DR TB. However, despite innovations in TB treatment, uptake of new regimens has been limited and the lengthy timeline involved in implementing new regimens has been challenging. Before implementing new regimens, some countries require locally generated evidence, which extends the implementation timeline. The registration of new drugs and supply chain issues also present regimen implementation challenges globally. Advances toward shorter regimens and countries' increasing interest in TB research are potential opportunities to be leveraged in the TB therapeutic space, he noted. Prior to the COVID-19 pandemic, global progress was being made toward achieving the United Nations High-Level Meeting targets for TB treatment for 2018–2022 (see Figure 3-1) (WHO, 2020).

Overview of the Global Burden of Drug-Resistant Tuberculosis in 2021

Zignol summarized major issues related to the global burden of DR TB as the COVID-19 pandemic continued through 2021. The global status of TB control has worsened because of the COVID-19 pandemic, and it will continue to worsen as the pandemic continues. He emphasized that DR TB is a major global health threat, but limited data are available to develop accurate projections of global DR TB trends. While absolute numbers of TB cases are decreasing, the proportion of DR TB is increasing. Current TB and DR TB testing practices and technologies are not sufficient, underscoring the urgent need for a POC TB test. Advances in research and practice have brought about more treatment regimens than have ever been available before—with many regimens shorter than ever

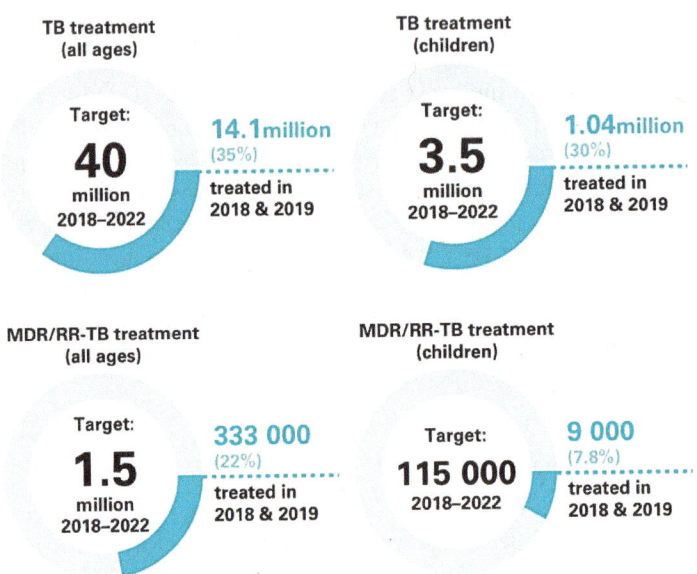

FIGURE 3-1 Progress toward 2018–2022 global targets for the number of people treated for tuberculosis.
SOURCES: Zignol presentation, September 14, 2021; WHO, 2020.

before—yet new regimen uptake is slow in many countries, meaning that significant progress must be made quickly in order to reach the 2018–2022 global TB treatment targets.

Discussion

Noting that the uptake by countries of new WHO recommendations on TB control is often slow, Ditiu asked about the slow pace of diagnostic development and the slow uptake of treatment regimens. Zignol cited supply chain constraints as a barrier to uptake. Manufacturers are often uninterested in investing in TB control products, particularly products for interventions that will ultimately benefit a relatively small number of patients. Countries' preference for locally generated evidence is another factor, noted Zignol. A country that wants to replicate a study that has been conducted elsewhere may delay the implementation of a new regimen by 5 years or more. International coordination and convincing leaders of the reliability of global evidence could help to shorten the implementation timeline. Involving stakeholders from various countries in the planning of initial research efforts could also help to streamline the implementation process.

RAPID ACCELERATION OF DIAGNOSTICS TECHNOLOGY: COVID-19 PANDEMIC EXPERIENCE

Presented by Matthew McMahon, National Institutes of Health

McMahon discussed efforts to rapidly accelerate the development of diagnostic technology for COVID-19 and highlighted lessons learned that could potentially be applied to TB diagnostics. He explained that the Rapid Acceleration of Diagnostics Technology program (RADx) is a large collaborative initiative to speed innovation in developing, commercializing, and implementing innovative approaches and technologies for COVID-19 testing.[1] RADx was established in 2020, when the U.S. National Institutes of Health (NIH) allocated an unprecedented $1.5 billion to expand and optimize the performance of COVID-19 testing technologies, $500 million of which was channeled to RADx via the National Institute of Biomedical Imaging and Bioengineering. RADx was built and layered upon the Point-of-Care Technologies Research Network (POCTRN)[2] (see Box 3-2) with the aims of expanding the number of, type of, and access to COVID-19 testing technologies and optimizing performance by aligning those testing technologies with community needs. POCTRN, like other proof-of-concept centers funded by NIH, combines and coordinates expertise from basic science communities and commercial stakeholders. This kind of cross-sectoral collaborative approach is fundamental to delivering innovative diagnostic technology into the hands of users, said McMahon.

Rapid Acceleration of Diagnostics Technology Innovation Funnel

McMahon described how RADx's technology innovation funnel process was designed to advance COVID-19 diagnostics. The innovation funnel process was intended to rapidly identify and evaluate narrowly targeted proposals by first filtering all applications through an initial viability evaluation to identify the most promising technologies. Next, during the deep-dive (or "Shark Tank") phase, a panel of technical and business experts worked intensively with proposers for a week to more comprehensively evaluate their proposed plans and ideas. Based on the deep-dive exercises, the first-phase awardees were selected to receive the first tranche of funding to conduct tech-

---

[1] More information about RADx is available at https://www.nih.gov/research-training/medical-research-initiatives/radx (accessed October 20, 2021).

[2] More information about the Point-of-Care Technologies Research Network is available at https://www.poctrn.org (accessed October 20, 2021).

> **BOX 3-2**
> **Point-of-Care Technologies Research Network**
>
> The Point-of-Care Technologies Research Network (POCTRN) is an existing network of proof-of-concept centers formed in 2007 to drive the development of point-of-care (POC) diagnostic technologies through collaborative efforts across government, academia, and industry to merge scientific and technical capabilities with clinical need. With the network hub as a coordinating center, POCTRN draws upon resources and unique expertise at four satellite centers—Georgia Institute of Technology/Emory University, Johns Hopkins University, Northwestern University, and University of Massachusetts. The network had been developing diagnostic testing solutions since 2007, so when the COVID-19 pandemic emerged in 2020, POCTRN was immediately activated to inject funding and expertise toward developing COVID-19 diagnostics. As part of this effort, three new core components were added to the network: a validation core, a clinical studies core, and a deployment core. Each of these cores brings extensive industry expertise to bear on the challenges of COVID-19 diagnostics, with more than 900 experts and contributors from government, academic, and industrial sectors participating in the project. As of September 2020, the validation core had completed more than 60 projects with over 2,500 total participants. The clinical studies core focuses on designing trials and developing digital health platforms under the auspices of a single institutional review board. The deployment core focuses on supply chains, manufacturing, and user communities.
>
> SOURCES: Presented by Matthew McMahon on September 14, 2021; https://www.poctrn.org.

nology validation, prototype development, and other initial work to prepare for the next phase of funding for manufacturing scale-up.

In the first two rounds of innovation funnels (2020–2021), RADx received more than 800 applications—mostly from small businesses, but also from academic groups, start-up companies, and mid- and large-sized businesses—and 35 projects received major funding from initial product development to manufacturing scale-up. These projects included a wide range of diagnostic innovations, including POC and home-use diagnostic products, laboratory diagnostic tools, and laboratory products. A primary aim of the project was to accelerate the validation of emerging technologies, including next-generation technologies such as CRISPR and nanoparticle applications, noted McMahon. RADx funded the development of the first commercially available home-use COVID-19 diagnostic test in the United States, developed by Ellume.[3] This home-use diagnostic tool used nanotechnology, mak-

---

[3] More information about Ellume is available at https://www.ellumehealth.com (accessed October 21, 2021).

ing its rapid advancement from technological validation to emergency use authorization and commercial availability especially noteworthy.

Impact Effect of Rapid Acceleration of Diagnostics Technology Projects

McMahon described the impact of RADx projects as of July 2021.[4] Cumulatively, RADx projects brought 667 million COVID-19 tests to market between September 2020 and July 2021, creating a COVID-19 diagnostic capacity equivalent to approximately 5 million tests per day. RADx has helped to secure 28 emergency use authorizations, including three for home-use tests and the first emergency use authorization for an over-the-counter COVID-19 diagnostic product. Furthermore, RADx has secured $1.1 billion from special congressional authorizations and $1.3 billion in private capital to support more than 100 companies since its inception.

"Say Yes! COVID Test" Program

McMahon highlighted RADx's collaboration with the U.S. Centers for Disease Control and Prevention and the "Say Yes! COVID Test" program. This collaboration was aimed at delivering COVID-19 tests to those in underserved communities and in areas with high levels of social vulnerability.[5] As of September 2021, the program had delivered 2 million home-use tests in numerous U.S. cities. The program was designed to assess the efficacy and effectiveness of providing home-use tests 2–3 times per week. The program's outcome measures included SARS-CoV-2 prevalence and incidence, percentage of test positivity by volume, community cell phone mobility, and wastewater surveillance. The program also provided participants with an optional digital assistant that provided reminders and instructions, offered test interpretation and guidance for positive test results, and reported results to state agencies in Michigan and Tennessee.

While the "Say Yes! COVID Test" program has been effective in delivering tests to individuals in need, various challenges have been encountered, said McMahon. For instance, it is difficult to ensure that individuals who receive tests actually use them, and it is even more difficult to ensure that they are used serially to maintain surveillance. Additionally, there were concerns that some individuals may discontinue adhering to public health or medical guidelines upon receiving a negative COVID-19 test result—mean-

---

[4] More information about the impact of RADx is available at https://www.nibib.nih.gov/covid-19/radx-tech-program/radx-tech-dashboard (accessed October 21, 2021).

[5] More information about the "Say Yes! Covid Test" program is available at https://sayyescovidtest.org/ (accessed October 21, 2021), and https://www.healthaffairs.org/do/10.1377/forefront.20211025.437195 (accessed January 28, 2022).

ing that persons who test negative may discontinue quarantine practices or fail to follow up with health care providers. Such challenges demonstrate that technological innovation alone is not sufficient to address complex disease control challenges; social science, behavioral economics, and other disciplines must be involved in public health interventions. McMahon cited COVID-19 vaccine hesitancy as a prime example. The rapid development and distribution of messenger RNA (mRNA) vaccines were not sufficient to ensure maximal uptake of vaccines among U.S. or world populations, as vaccine hesitancy has stymied progress in vaccination rates, even in settings with ample vaccine supply.

Leveraging the Digital Health Infrastructure

Strengthening and leveraging the digital health infrastructure can facilitate linkages between diagnostic innovations, health systems, and health surveillance, said McMahon. For instance, providing home-use COVID-19 tests to individuals is valuable for the recipient, but these products have far greater effect if test results are connected to health and surveillance systems. In addition to developing and testing reporting standards for certain COVID-19 home-use tests, there are ongoing efforts to use the digital health infrastructure by providing incentives for people to use the at-home tests and connecting test users with health care providers after testing is complete. Mobile phone applications can be used to (1) provide users with testing instructions, (2) interpret test strip results using machine learning, (3) conduct surveys to screen users for symptoms, and (4) connect users' data to data hubs for use in reporting, collecting state and federal data, validating health passes, and contact tracing. Because many diagnostic tools can be linked to public health systems in valuable ways, the RADx deployment core assists every RADx project in optimizing its use of the digital health infrastructure.

Lessons for Tuberculosis Control

McMahon highlighted several factors that have contributed to the success of the program and could be applied to TB control efforts: (1) obtaining a large-scale dedicated financial commitment made funding immediately accessible; (2) building upon existing programmatic infrastructure allowed for the rapid launch of the program within mere days of receipt of funding; (3) fostering direct, focused interagency collaboration, particularly with Food and Drug Administration (FDA), Centers for Disease Control and Prevention, and other partners; and (4) focusing intently on commercial viability.

Interagency collaboration has been invaluable to the success of RADx, said McMahon. For instance, FDA collaboration was vital for rapidly advancing RADx technologies from development to emergency use authorization and commercial rollout. Weekly meetings between stakeholders from RADx and FDA's in vitro diagnostics team were held to provide FDA with early previews of forthcoming and often novel technologies being developed through the initiative. RADx stakeholders used these meetings to establish a detailed understanding of the dynamic regulatory landscape, to inform the design of validation studies to address FDA's concerns, and to streamline the authorization process. The Biomedical Advanced Research and Development Authority (BARDA) and various Department of Defense programs provided funding and support for rapid manufacturing scale-up of newly developed diagnostic tools.

McMahon also emphasized the importance of RADx's narrow focus on ensuring commercial viability and bringing diagnostic tools to market as fast as possible. In the early months of RADx, White House leadership and the Department of Health and Homeland Security demanded frequent progress updates with a specific focus on test production and distribution status. This pressure to deliver commercially viable products to market was challenging for RADx leadership; however, this top-down focus on commercially viable products was instrumental in bringing about ground-breaking technological innovations. During the early phases of RADx, expert stakeholders were conducting multiple efforts in parallel: rapidly validating technologies, developing benchtop assays into prototypes, navigating the regulatory landscape, and gathering knowledge of distribution and supply chain needs for forthcoming diagnostic products. Despite the successes of RADx, McMahon acknowledged that much work remains to be done to improve COVID-19 testing capacity in the United States.

Ongoing Challenges and the Future of RADx

McMahon discussed RADx's ongoing challenges and potential future applications of the model. Maintaining and monitoring the COVID-19 reporting infrastructure has been a major challenge since the onset of the pandemic (Banco, 2021). Furthermore, it has been difficult for public health officials to detect and quickly react to hotspots. Insufficient screening and surveillance—particularly in high-risk settings such as schools and long-term care facilities—has compounded these challenges (Geske, 2021; Vigdor, 2021). It has also been challenging to deliver simple, fast, and affordable POC testing solutions to those most in need.

In the future, the RADx process and networks will be used to address diagnostic needs for other pathogens and promote disease control preparedness, said McMahon. RADx is focusing on four pillars going forward:

1. Facilitating real-time data collection by modernizing and expanding digital health infrastructure and reporting systems to integrate

diagnostic results from laboratory tests, POC tests, and over-the-counter tests;
2. Expanding access to better rapid tests by using the disruptive power of e-commerce and direct-to-consumer practices to distribute over-the-counter and POC diagnostic tools and report results;
3. Developing multiplex POC and laboratory tests for differential diagnostics, such as a single multiplex test to detect SARS-CoV-2, influenza A/B, and respiratory syncytial virus;[6] and
4. Enabling fast, accurate, and cost-effective surveillance that includes genetic sequencing to track variances in diseases across populations (e.g., using new laboratory and POC diagnostics tools to collect genotyping and informatics data; wastewater surveillance).

Discussion

Gail Cassell, senior lecturer on global health and social medicine at Harvard Medical School, asked whether TB might be well suited for addition into a multiplex test or whether standalone tests would be preferable for detecting TB. McMahon replied that multiplex tests could be used to detect TB, but the current global focus on COVID-19 has limited the scope of funding for such projects—for instance, all RADx funding is part of a larger allocation that is narrowly focused on the COVID-19 response. However, RADx has prioritized the development of platforms and multiplex technologies to facilitate the adaptation of new COVID-19 diagnostic tools to other pathogens in the future. Given the urgency to develop new TB diagnostic tools, Cassell asked whether it would be more prudent to forge ahead with standalone TB diagnostic research or to try to integrate advances in TB diagnostics into efforts to develop a respiratory multiplex assay that might be supported through COVID-19 response funding. She emphasized the potential benefits of a respiratory multiplex assay that could detect TB, COVID-19, influenza, and perhaps community-acquired pneumonia infections. McMahon said that numerous organizations are funding multiplex testing research—including BARDA. The narrow focus of RADx helped to catalyze funding and attention, thus TB diagnostic research could benefit from similarly focused efforts, he suggested.

Mansoura asked about the sustainability of RADx's efforts—given how quickly the capacity for COVID-19 testing has accelerated and expanded worldwide—and how to use those efforts most effectively to address more

---

[6] McMahon pointed out that including COVID-19 testing in multiplex tests would present regulatory challenges. This is because COVID-19 tests are being approved under emergency use authorization, while other tests would likely be subject to the standard regulatory environment.

persistent diagnostic demands. She also asked about the constraints posed by temporary single-disease funding (e.g., during the Middle East respiratory syndrome coronavirus [MERS-Cov] and Ebola virus disease outbreaks). McMahon responded that RADx tries to select platform technologies that have the potential to be applied to other infectious diseases in order to achieve long-term sustainability. Ideally, partnerships forged in response to the COVID-19 pandemic will be able to flex and pivot rapidly, perhaps with government assistance, to new and forthcoming challenges as they arise.

Vo noted that the availability of disease-specific funding can influence research agendas. For instance, Ceres Nanosciences was supported by RADx during the COVID-19 pandemic; prior to the pandemic, the company was developing technologies for TB control. He asked how the rapid incubation model employed by RADx can be applied in fields with less funding, such as TB. McMahon said that the RADx model has been thoroughly studied so that it can be applied to future research needs. Further, he speculated that it may be possible to secure funding to replicate a RADx-like project aimed at TB diagnostics.

ADVANCES IN TUBERCULOSIS DIAGNOSTICS

Point-of-Care Molecular Platform for Diagnosis of Tuberculosis and Other Infectious Respiratory Diseases

Presented by Morten Ruhwald, FIND

Ruhwald presented on POC molecular platforms for diagnosis of tuberculosis and other infectious respiratory diseases. He commended advances in research and innovation achieved during the COVID-19 pandemic, highlighting the flexibility demonstrated by regulatory, political, and manufacturing stakeholders and the advances in manufacturing occurring in LMICs. However, the growing install base and integrated COVID-19 response from clinics and laboratories has come at the expense of certain TB control efforts.[7] Moving forward, he suggested focusing on building back and expanding TB control capacity by building upon advances brought forth by the COVID-19 response, such as the expansion of digital health infrastructures and innovations in self-sampling and home-use tests. For TB control efforts to adapt to the new disease control landscape, TB control programs will need to break out of their silos, he said. Moreover, manufacturers will need incentives to develop new TB diagnostic tools and platform technolo-

---

[7] The term "install base" refers to the number of units of a product that is in use. See https://www.credenceresearch.com/info/installed-base-scenario-medical-devices (accessed February 25, 2022).

gies by pivoting the newly developed footprint for COVID-19 diagnostics to explore simultaneous or bidirectional testing. The complexity of sputum testing is a pressing challenge in TB diagnostics, he said. Efforts are underway to develop simpler tongue-swab or urine-based diagnostic technologies and to explore the use of face masks or other strategies for capturing aerosol samples for diagnostic testing. He added that from the developers' perspective, it would be helpful to shorten the length of clinical trials and facilitate the assessment of multiple technologies in parallel. TB diagnostics and control still rely largely upon older tools and analog reporting technology. To advance TB diagnostics and control into the digital age, he suggested using advances in POC diagnostic tools and data-tracking dashboards that have emerged in response to the COVID-19 pandemic.

Innovations for Tackling Tuberculosis in the Time of COVID-19

Presented by Zvi Marom and Eran Zahavy, BATM

Marom and Zahavy discussed BATM Advanced Communications' innovative approach to tackling TB amid the COVID-19 pandemic. Its approach is to focus on substantially reducing the cost of diagnostic testing and to initiate TB treatment rapidly after an accurate diagnosis, including the diagnosis of antibiotic resistance in the same test. It is currently developing a new test to detect MDR/XDR TB that uses a combinatoric algorithm scanning system,[8] which can be used for population screening at very low cost. The system can be used to run diagnostic tests for multiple respiratory diseases simultaneously (e.g., TB, COVID-19, influenza, pneumonia) in a single plate, with test results directly reported to digitized patient medical records. Based on modeling simulations of TB testing in Uganda, this system could potentially process more than 4,000 samples per day, reducing reagent costs by a factor of between 8 and 10 and enabling rapid testing of an entire country's population.

The next step in the development process is to replace classical polymerase chain reaction (PCR) diagnostics with isothermal technology, said Marom. The isothermal single test is a diagnostic platform for conducting rapid, easy-to-use, saliva-based, molecular diagnostic screening for various indications. This disruptive, modular, and scalable approach is implementable in settings without access to laboratory services; it yields results within minutes that are even more precise than highly reliable lateral flow tests. Isothermal testing has already been used for COVID-19 diagnosis and

---

[8] More information about BATM Advanced Communications' molecular diagnostic test for TB is available at https://www.batm.com/rns-rnr/posts/2021/march/batm-develops-molecular-diagnostics-test-for-tuberculosis (accessed October 25, 2021).

could be adapted for new indications and targets. For instance, isothermal tests for TB diagnostics could be scaled up for deployment within 18 months, he said.

Marom compared BATM Advanced Communications' isothermal system, called rolling circle amplification (RCA), with PCR diagnostic methods. RCA is qualitative—but will soon be quantitative—and is at least as sensitive and specific as PCR, but provides results within 25 minutes. The diagnostic system, called NATlab, is a fully automated, sample-to-answer system that provides multiplexed analysis of individual samples against 100 or more targets. If adapted for TB diagnosis, this technology could use a single sputum sample to diagnose TB, detect specific mutations to identify antibiotic resistance, and optimize patient treatment. Additionally, NATlab diagnostic devices harness Internet connectivity and AI to predict disease trends using diagnostic data; for example, NATlab diagnostic tools were used to predict and map the movement of the COVID-19 pandemic. Moreover, this platform-based diagnostic technology can be used to diagnose many diseases, including sexually transmitted diseases, meningitis, and others.

Improving X-ray Accessibility

Presented by Luan Vo, Friends for International Tuberculosis Relief

Vo described the implementation of ultraportable X-ray technology and the use of AI for X-ray interpretation for TB detection in Vietnam. He described how prior to the COVID-19 pandemic, around 170,000 people in Vietnam became sick with TB each year, but only 104,505 cases were treated—leaving approximately 65,000 untreated cases—and there were 11,400 TB-related deaths (WHO, 2020). To reduce the gap of untreated cases, Vietnam has used active case-finding techniques such as contact investigating, mobile mass screening, door-to-door screening, and seeking out vulnerable populations.

Vo compared the current standard for mobile X-ray with the new ultraportable X-ray technology that Vietnam began using in 2021. Currently, the trucks used for mobile X-ray screening weigh in excess of 2,000 kg and face significant logistical barriers. For example, to reach island populations, these X-ray trucks must be transported on freight ships. In contrast, new battery-operated, hand-held ultraportable X-ray devices are about the size of a camera and weigh only 3.5 kg. The extreme portability of these devices makes it possible to bring X-ray screening directly to the doorsteps of those most in need.

Early findings from a study comparing the new ultraportable X-ray system with conventional X-ray devices suggest that ultraportable X-ray systems can extend safe and reliable access to high-quality X-ray diagnostic services to vulnerable groups (Vo et al., 2021). Based on these promising findings, Vietnam has piloted the use of ultraportable X-ray devices for screening 800 people for TB in two sites: an island and a mountainous district with several villages that were home to ethnic minority populations. The devices performed as expected and detected many cases of TB, despite the pilot being conducted during the COVID-19 pandemic when health seeking was restricted. However, further process optimization will need to address current limitations of the devices. For instance, the battery life was suboptimal and could capture only 40 images per charge (which takes 4 hours); this could result in TB screening campaigns being reliant on grid-powered systems. The ultraportable X-ray devices could last for an entire day using large capacity backup batteries, but these required power switches as charging was not possible during operation, undermining both user experience and device portability. The screening campaign also faced connectivity challenges related to the wireless detector panels that connect to the X-ray device, with loss of Bluetooth connectivity frequently causing delays in image transfers to the interpretation station.

Vo and colleagues have also evaluated the use of multiple AI solutions to aid chest radiography interpretation during TB screening, finding that many AI solutions can detect TB with a high level of accuracy.[9] Vo shared that AI interpretations were on par with—or superior to—X-ray interpretations by intermediate radiologists (with 5 years or more of relevant experience), although none of the solutions were better at detecting TB than expert radiologists (30 years or more of relevant experience). The implementation results further suggest that AI interpretation could be used to triage out approximately 30 percent of non-TB X-rays with limited losses in sensitivity, thus saving radiologists' time by reducing the number of non-normal X-ray images they need to evaluate for potential TB cases. Although AI interpretation has the potential to decrease cost and increase operational effectiveness, the technology will need further calibration to address confounders that can undermine its accuracy, such as history of TB, age, and the radiography equipment used.

Implementation Challenges with New Tuberculosis Diagnostics

Presented by Kaiser Shen, United States Agency for International Development

Shen shared insights from his work at USAID on POC TB diagnostics, TB diagnostic networks, and implementation challenges. Although the pipeline for TB diagnostics is expanding, the forthcoming tools will not be suf-

---

[9] This study has been published since the time of the workshop; see Codlin et al., 2021.

ficient because they remain primarily sputum-based tests. He highlighted the need for investment in developing biomarker-based tests to detect individuals most at risk of developing TB. Diagnostic systems also rely upon support systems—such as specimen referral systems and diagnostic data connectivity—that are necessary to ensure the full expression of new diagnostic technologies. He predicted that as new technologies are developed, the countries that are most in need of new assays are likely to encounter challenges in absorbing and implementing these new technologies. TB diagnostics have traditionally been configured using a tiered system that focuses on top-down approaches, but the availability of POC TB diagnostic tools would transform this paradigm, said Shen. As older tools that were implemented within a top-down infrastructure are replaced by new technologies—as occurred with the rollout of GeneXpert—their accompanying infrastructures will need to be replaced as well.

Implementation challenges associated with TB diagnostics include difficulties with POC testing in remote and rural locations, where it is difficult to provide services and conduct equipment maintenance. Health care providers in remote or rural locations also face challenges related to unstable power supplies or lack of adequately trained staff. Improving visibility within networks is another challenge that will require large investment in collecting and reporting diagnostic data, particularly in settings with gaps between diagnosis and reporting. Moving forward, Shen suggested implementing new systems to improve data collection and reporting to drive uptake and sustainability. He also noted that some countries scaled up GeneXpert implementation too rapidly without using data to inform the placement of diagnostic equipment. As new technologies are developed and implemented, better understandings of existing data and data flow could help inform clinical, programmatic, and political decision making.

IMPROVING ADHERENCE, INFECTION CONTROL CAPACITIES, AND COST-EFFECTIVENESS

Integrated Community Response to the COVID-19 Pandemic in Karachi, Pakistan

Presented by Aamir Khan, IRD

Khan discussed the comprehensive approach to COVID-19 and TB testing implemented in Pakistan that adapted the Interactive Research and Development (IRD) model of integrated community response to TB control. When Pakistan's first COVID-19 surge began in March 2020 in Karachi—a large city center with a population of 20 million—a mass TB screening campaign was put in place using mobile X-ray vans. COVID-19 screening was integrated into the existing TB screening resources to aid in the pandemic response by offering combined TB and SARS-CoV-2 screening across the city. Individuals were offered PCR testing if they had symptoms or had been exposed to COVID-19. Between April and July 2020, more than 23,000 people in Karachi received combined screening, of whom 112 were diagnosed with TB and 6 were diagnosed with TB and COVID-19. Through various combinations of symptoms, exposure information, and X-ray screening, the efforts diagnosed 1,385 cases of COVID-19 via PCR testing.

Adapting the TB Screening System to Address COVID-19

The existing TB screening system was modified by adapting IRD's TB control model to address the high burden of COVID-19 in Karachi more directly, said Khan. IRD used its existing network of high school girls (i.e., *Kiran Sitaras*) trained to support TB control by having them promote mask use and handwashing in neighborhoods, screen households for potential cases of COVID-19, and distribute information. IRD engaged 200 mental health counselors to provide psychosocial support—for example, providing food packages and cash to patients in isolation and families in quarantine. They enlisted 200 contact tracers to locate all index patients, conduct a risk-based classification of contacts of confirmed COVID-19 patients, and track home-based quarantine using a mobile app and patient database. IRD also offered interventions to reduce COVID-19 stigma.

Khan explained that IRD had already been working with private providers in Karachi because it is the first line of care for many people with TB symptoms. Once IRD began shifting efforts toward the COVID-19 response, it worked with more than 1,000 private practitioners by offering training and equipping them with needed protective equipment, pulse oximeters, oxygen cylinders, and diagnostic referral links. Neighborhood clinics were able to triage COVID-19 cases, offering screening for symptoms, pulse oximetry, oxygen therapy, and oral or intravenous steroids. IRD also supported the provision of free X-ray diagnostics and oxygen therapy, as well as facilitated two-way referral between emergency rooms and isolation facilities. PCR and antibody COVID-19 testing were provided for a fee in the private sector, with PCR testing offered for free at certain public and nonprofit laboratories. IRD also systematically collected COVID-19 screening and treatment data throughout the community response to COVID-19.

Provision of Oxygen Therapy, COVID-19 Screening, and Phone-Based Contact Tracing

Khan provided an overview of efforts to provide oxygen therapy, conduct COVID-19 screening, and use phone-based contact tracing for COVID-

19 patients in Karachi. He emphasized that when setting up a city's capacity to provide oxygen therapy, relatively few additional resources are needed to ensure complete coverage throughout the entire city. With the appropriate motivation and forethought, IRD was able to create an oxygen supply network so that anyone in Karachi with difficulty breathing could access oxygen. Among those who received oxygen therapy between June 2020 and August 2021, 96 percent were sent home and tested for COVID-19 in the following days, averting unnecessary emergency room visits during the pandemic. Although the absolute effect of these oxygen therapy interventions was relatively small, they demonstrate the value of using existing TB infrastructure in responding to a pandemic, he added.

IRD's general practitioner network was instrumental to COVID-19 screening efforts in Karachi, said Khan. More than 47,000 presumptive-positive COVID-19 patients were screened at clinics in Karachi between June 2020 and July 2021. However, owing to limited testing access and the high cost of PCR testing in the private sector, a large proportion of patients were never tested for COVID-19 despite being presumptive positive and symptomatic (82 percent) or presumptive positive with subsided symptoms (99 percent).

Phone-Based Contact Tracing Among Patients Who Tested Positive for COVID-19

IRD realigned its existing TB contact-tracing team and system to conduct COVID-19 contact tracing, identifying almost 23,000 index patients, of whom about 16,000 were contacted. More than 7,300 reported untested contacts. This contact-tracing effort was the only method by which data were collected regarding the outcomes for patients with positive PCR tests—1 percent of the index patients had died, and 55 percent had recovered. Between April 2020 and April 2021, 128 patients who had tested positive for COVID-19 died in Karachi. Most deaths among those with positive PCR tests occurred within the first 2 weeks after testing positive and most died in health facilities, but many died at home after testing positive for COVID-19. Khan surmised that these deaths probably would not have been reported if not for the contact-tracing efforts. This is another example of the value of an existing TB infrastructure for COVID-19 response, said Khan.

Lessons Learned from Adapting Integrated Community Response to COVID-19 in Karachi

Khan highlighted lessons learned from Karachi's COVID-19 experience and IRD's adaptation of existing TB systems to manage the pandemic surge. A COVID-19 surge can quickly overwhelm any active TB screening system.

In Karachi, for example, there were about 10-fold more COVID-19 patients than TB patients in the first X-ray screening campaign. Thus, mass antigen rapid diagnostic testing will be key for addressing COVID-19 surges in the future. Such testing is now being supported by existing TB partners, including FIND and Stop TB. Khan emphasized that previous investments in TB control have supported the COVID-19 pandemic response, as demonstrated by the preexistence of a functional TB screening system that enabled Karachi's initial COVID-19 response. Moreover, Karachi's initial pandemic response was bolstered by the existing TB contact-tracing systems, mental health support systems, private-sector provider networks, and data-collecting and -reporting systems.

Telehealth and Digital Adherence Technologies

Presented by Bruce Thomas, The Arcady Group

Thomas discussed how DATs can facilitate differentiated and virtual care for persons affected by TB. Despite the fact that TB is treatable and curable, too few patients successfully traverse the TB care cascade from infection to successful treatment. For instance, a study evaluating TB treatment cascades in India and South Africa found that the proportion of individuals who completed each step of the TB care cascade progressively declined (Subbaraman et al., 2016). From burden to testing, diagnosis, treatment initiation, treatment completion, notification, and treatment success/recurrence-free survival, individuals fell off the care cascade at each step. He noted that the care cascade outcomes are often worse for patients with MDR TB or TB with HIV.[10]

Effect of the COVID-19 Pandemic on Global Tuberculosis Control

Thomas described the extent to which the COVID-19 pandemic has worsened global TB control. Overall, approximately 1 million fewer persons affected by TB were tested and treated in 2020 than in 2019, representing an 18 percent decline (Global Fund, 2021). During that time, the number of persons on treatment for MDR TB and XDR TB declined by 19 percent and 37 percent, respectively. Among those with HIV and TB, the number of persons on both antiretroviral treatment and TB treatment declined by 16 percent. Despite these challenges, the pandemic has had some limited

---

[10] Thomas shared the statistics that in India, only 41 percent of MDR TB cases were diagnosed, with only 11 percent of those achieving recurrence-free survival, and in South Africa, 82 percent of patients with HIV and TB co-infection were diagnosed, and 52 percent of those achieved treatment success.

favorable effects on TB treatment and control. For example, the COVID-19 pandemic has accelerated the trend of giving TB patients custody of their own medications, and patients self-administering their TB medications has become far more common. TB programs have also increasingly taken advantage of digital tools—such as telehealth and digital adherence monitoring—to bring TB services to the people and communities in need. These trends are expected to outlast the COVID-19 pandemic and strengthen efforts to fight other diseases, he added. According to a letter from the executive director in the Global Fund's *Results Report 2021*:

> COVID-19 has catalyzed a multitude of innovations across all three diseases, such as multi-month dispensing of TB and HIV drugs; using digital tools to monitor TB treatment or enhance prevention interventions; and introducing patient-centered diagnostic approaches, such as co-testing for HIV, TB and COVID-19. Many of these innovations will outlast the crisis and strengthen our fight against HIV, TB, and malaria. (Global Fund, 2021)

Differentiated Care Through Integrated Digital Adherence Technologies

Thomas discussed the challenges in TB treatment adherence and the potential benefits of DATs, which have particular value in the context of the COVID-19 pandemic. Adherence is a multifactor behavioral issue that changes over time. Poor adherence in TB treatment can be attributed to various factors such as the prevalence of long and complicated treatment regimens, confusion about dosing, treatment side effects, and the use of a directly observed therapy–short course. The last factor is known to be stigmatizing, burdensome, and inconsistent with many patients' lifestyles. Poor adherence is known to be associated with TB recurrence (Thomas et al., 2005), making adherence critical for success in TB treatment. Their 2005 study found a strong relationship between adherence and post-treatment TB recurrence; recurrence rates for very irregular adherence were found to be 25 percent (Thomas et al., 2005). A 2018 meta-analysis found that TB patients taking shortened regimens with less than 90 percent adherence had a 5.6 times increased risk of recurrence (Imperial et al., 2018).

Integrated DATs are being developed to support TB patients while capturing their dosage histories, said Thomas. These technologies have been designed to be affordable, scalable, TB-appropriate, and accessible to patients in high-TB-burden regions through the use of phones and other available technological platforms. Importantly, these technologies are integrated such that a single system can be used to assign DATs to any patient and allow providers to access and review compiled dosing histories. These technologies also offer patients and providers choices so they can select the tools that best fit patients' lifestyles and treatment regimens.

Thomas presented several examples of integrated DATs. 99DOTS uses augmented packaging to reveal codes as a person takes their medications,[11] and users report their dose adherences using a toll-free call or SMS. Video-observed therapy can also be used in lieu of directly observed therapies by allowing patients to share videos of themselves taking their medications, which can be reviewed by health care workers to understand their patients' adherence. Various forms of "smart pillboxes" contain electronic components that remind patients to take their treatments and send signals reporting adherence when the box is opened. The Everwell Hub is an open-source digital platform that allows providers to register patients, allocate them to specific DATs, and review data such as historical adherence.

Thomas presented a model for using DATs to provide differentiated and virtual care (Subbaraman et al., 2018). Differentiated care refers to providing different intensities and types of care based on a patient's level of medication adherence as measured by the DAT. In this model, DATs provide self-administering patients with reminders and dosing assistance. DATs can be used to electronically observe or verify daily dosing, to deliver detailed dosing histories to health systems, and to apply evidence-based escalation protocols. Dosing histories are used to continuously triage patients and identify nonadherent patients, who can be prioritized for engagement by providers to understand and assess reasons for poor adherence (e.g., experiencing side effects, needing refill, being asymptomatic). He also presented an example of a patient adherence timeline, which detailed a patient's treatment adherence over time, including treatment registration, medication receipt, automated patient reminders and adherence, instances of patient non-adherence, health staff interventions, and overall adherence at the time of treatment completion.

The rationale for using a DAT-enabled differential care approach is strong, said Thomas. These approaches reduce the burden on patients and empower them to manage their treatments unless they have demonstrable adherence issues. These approaches are also transparent—giving patients and providers equal access to patients' dosing history—and thus promote trust between patients and providers. They shift the perception of adherence measurement to be similar to other vital signs. Health systems gain behavioral insights into dosing histories to highlight unique patient-specific patterns of non-adherence. Additionally, these approaches enable and inform patient–provider discussions about adherence challenges and the specific steps patients can take to address those challenges. He added that DAT approaches are approved by WHO based on favorable results from a range of trials conducted in the United States, European Union, and high-burden regions. For

---

[11] More information about 99DOTS is available at 99dots.org (accessed November 3, 2021).

instance, one study found that DATs significantly improved adherence among antiretroviral therapy patients in China (Sabin et al., 2010).

Thomas described progress in building a strong evidence base for DAT in clinical trials and implementing DAT in clinical practice between 2015 and 2020, prior to the COVID-19 pandemic, leading to WHO's approval. The process began with a catalytic innovation phase to develop DAT tool kits, followed by a proof-of-concept phase with evaluations conducted in India and China. WHO then issued supportive guidance for DATs, and TB Resource Group for Advocacy and Community Health grants funded the implementation of 13 projects across 11 countries. During the subsequent transition to scale phase, funded by Unitaid, DATs were scaled up to more than 70,000 patients. In 2020, the Global Fund began providing multiyear support for DATs in approximately 13 countries, and continued phases of innovation since 2020 have been led by Global Health Labs and the Bill & Melinda Gates Medical Research Institute.

Effect of COVID-19 on Digital Adherence Technologies

Thomas highlighted lessons learned from the implementation of DATs and ways that the COVID-19 pandemic has improved the DAT landscape. DATs are relatively affordable, readily scalable, and generally well accepted by patients and providers. However, lack of health care provider contact can cause patients to disengage from DATs. To address this issue, DATs provide escalation-based task lists to providers to help facilitate essential patient engagement and follow-up. When implemented properly, patients see their DAT as a direct connection to their provider, which encourages them to use DAT tools to facilitate that connection—for example, to use e-prescribing and refills or to ask questions about facility operations, dosing, side effects, or direct benefit transfer.

The COVID-19 pandemic provided an opportunity for DAT tool kits to be used to provide more virtual and at-home care in areas with limited access to health care facilities. DAT tool kits were rapidly adapted to address arising needs and to support virtual care. While DAT tool kits originally focused exclusively on adherence monitoring, they now offer patient-facing applications that provide patients with access to a wealth of information about their treatments, adherence, and overall care. These applications help to facilitate real-time virtual engagement between patients and providers. For instance, the Everwell Hub Health companion application and India's TB Aarogya Sathi application provide these features to patients around the world.

Thomas described advances in video observation technology, emphasizing that video observation can be useful for more than just dose monitoring. For instance, it can be used to facilitate asynchronous observation. Patients can use smartphones to record medication ingestion, and then health care workers can asynchronously view and record their observations via encrypted video. In addition to functioning as a standalone adherence system, this technology can be used as part of an integrated DAT approach using a digital platform (e.g., Everwell Hub). Video observation technology can also be used in clinical trials and in clinical practice. In response to the COVID-19 pandemic, SureAdhere, a video observation technology platform, has added two-way secure messaging to its platform, and soon its platform will offer live teleconsultations via video web conferencing.

The COVID-19 pandemic has accelerated a shift toward at-home care for persons affected by TB, said Thomas. It has fostered an unprecedented willingness to consider approaches other than facility-based care and tools, with existing DATs being used to foster a new model of at-home care that (1) allows patients to self-administer drugs with remote monitoring, (2) provides patients with dosing support and other support, (3) facilitates dose-history-informed differentiated care, (4) integrates diagnostics to support a "test and treat" model, and (5) fosters patient–provider engagement as virtual care increases. He was optimistic that TB care would not revert to the pre-pandemic condition and that many persons affected by TB will not be restricted to facility-based care in the future.

Innovative Strategies to Synergize Investments in Health Care Systems

Presented by Monique K. Mansoura, MITRE

Mansoura explored innovative strategies to synergize investments in health care systems with a focus on whether cancer and TB care can protect against pandemics. "TB is a natural partner in our efforts to better prepare for and protect populations against pandemics, while we are also building critical infrastructure for cancer and TB," she remarked. Various synergies at the molecular and health systems levels could be leveraged across TB, cancer, and pandemic events and allow for the whole health system to be improved, but such synergistic surpluses are not possible without deliberate action, meaningful measures, and checks to ensure accountability. Meaningful measures and accountabilities also help to build credibility with donors and investors, as well as incentivizing and rewarding innovations in flex competence, which Mansoura defined as the ability for a system's components and resources to be deployed to various efforts depending on changing needs. Through sustained commitments from leadership, governments, and investors, these synergies can improve care and preparedness. Mansoura maintained that TB and cancer care are naturally aligned in the effort to build a stronger critical infrastructure to support pandemic preparedness.

DETECTION

Mansoura emphasized the importance of a systems approach to the provision of care. A systems approach recognizes the roles of facilities, staff and workforce, and the materials and equipment that are all necessary to provide comprehensive care. Such an approach is key for leveraging synergies and achieving benefits, cost-effectiveness, and building capacity. A primary challenge in global health security is persistence in building capacity and the maintenance of sustained commitments. Investments that are more broadly targeted—investments that target more than one disease—help to maintain such a sustained commitment, she added.

Matrix of Preparedness and Event Occurrence

To discuss challenges related to preparedness for potential pandemics and health attacks, Mansoura presented an outcomes matrix showing potential outcomes based on the combination of event occurrences and preparedness (see Figure 3-2). COVID-19 is an example of a "horrible scenario" wherein a pandemic has occurred while preparedness measures were in place, yet they were inadequate to prevent immense loss of life and livelihood—although the consequences of the pandemic would have undoubtedly been even worse if no preparedness measures were in place at all. Mansoura emphasized the tenuousness of the "second guessing" outcome, wherein investments are made in preparedness but no attacks or pandemics occur, so there is continual second guessing about why that money was spent. For instance, no coronavirus vaccine was developed after SARS outbreaks in the early 2000s, nor was a vaccine developed in response to the MERS outbreak

Pandemic / Attack Occurs	Necessary Pandemic / Attack Preparedness	
+	+	A horrible scenario
+	-	The worst scenario*
-	+	2nd guessing
-	-	The dream outcome

FIGURE 3-2 Preparedness framework.
* U.S. government programs, such as BioShield, the Biomedical Advanced Research and Development Authority, and the Public Health Emergency Medical Countermeasures Enterprise were designed to prevent worst-case scenarios.
SOURCES: Mansoura presentation.

in 2012. She suggested that this failure to follow up was caused by second guessing of the investment in preparedness during times in which no immediate threat was present. Second guessing about preparedness for events that have not occurred is a "persistent paralyzer," said Mansoura. However, she continued, there is no reason to doubt that attacks and pandemics will occur in the future, so the "dream outcome" of no pandemics and a total lack of preparation should not be considered a realistic option. Synergistic investment in more persistent health spaces, such as TB and cancer, can help to address the barriers caused by second guessing. Moreover, the capacity developed through these investments can be leveraged in times of need to respond to attacks or pandemics, she added.

Current State of Global Cancer Care

Mansoura described the work of the International Cancer Expert Corps (ICEC) to transform global cancer care, reduce mortality, and improve the quality of life for people with cancer in LMICs and underserved regions worldwide through catalytic and disruptive innovation. Currently, underserved populations lack access to cancer care experts. Mansoura shared that while there is a surge of interest in the developed world to deliver high-quality cancer care, the current global health care environment encourages the depletion of talent (via brain drain) in LMICs. ICEC mentoring programs are designed to match experts with global needs through partnership programs and matched funding to support participants. ICEC helps to transform cancer care by partnering with local communities to build sustainable infrastructure and programs. Innovation in cancer care equipment is another pressing concern for ICEC. Radioactive cobalt-60 machines present environmental and security risks, and these devices lack the sophistication needed for modern radiotherapy. Additionally, there is no practical, accessible, and affordable technology available to meet global cancer care needs. ICEC is promoting innovation in equipment design by working to convene and engage stakeholders in the radiotherapy equipment design sector.

Achieving Health Systems with Flexible Competence

"Flexible competence" can be achieved by bridging the investment dichotomy between cancer and infectious diseases such as TB, suggested Mansoura. Overlaying the hotspots for infectious diseases and disease burdens for noncommunicable diseases reveals clear geographic alignment (Coleman et al., 2020). The control of both infectious diseases and noncommunicable diseases requires early detection and rapid response, and thus building capacity and capability in those areas will have multiple benefits. Convergent, adaptable medical care capacity building is a cost-effective and necessary approach for improving care for both infectious and noncommunicable disease, as both disease types have similar etiology and systemic responses (e.g., infectious agents, immunology, and inflammation).

Mansoura and colleagues have developed a model for dual-capacity health systems with flex competence that improves outcomes and preparedness for infectious diseases, including pandemics and TB, and noncommunicable diseases such as cancer (Coleman et al., 2020). The model highlights the interrelationships between noncommunicable diseases and infectious diseases. For instance, some cancers are caused by infectious diseases, and cancer patients are often susceptible to infection. Both disease groups can benefit from rapid, population-level assessment, which is a foundational capacity both for pandemic response, and ongoing prevention and treatment. Both disease groups require similar health care capacity for physical examination, laboratory and molecular diagnostics, diagnostic imaging, treatment and recurrence prevention, and modulation to address immune response and inflammation. An integrated health care system could offer flex competence in areas applicable across infectious diseases, noncommunicable diseases, pandemics, and disasters:

- Prevention of infectious diseases and immunization;
- Population surveillance;
- Prevention of noncommunicable diseases (e.g., screening, healthy lifestyle promotion, diet);
- Diagnostic capacity;
- Treatment, including palliative care; and
- Patient surveillance.

Ideally, these components would be built into an integrated health care system with the capacity to flex to address a range of disease types—including TB, COVID-19, and cancer—to improve health outcomes and strengthen preparedness.

Mansoura explained that the concept of flex competence refers to a health care system's adaptability to changing needs (Coleman et al., 2020). A high degree of flexibility and adaptability enables common health care capacities and resources to be continually evaluated and adapted based on need; leaders can then deputize these tested resources to where they are most needed. For instance, a health system may typically focus on noncommunicable diseases while maintaining baseline pandemic surveillance and infectious disease control efforts. However, in an early outbreak, that system might reduce noncommunicable disease capacity and shift its focus to pandemic surveillance and infectious disease control. On the other hand, a well-vaccinated community might focus more resources on noncommunicable diseases while maintaining reduced pandemic surveillance and infectious disease efforts.

Measuring Flex Competence

Mansoura presented metrics that can be applied to measure the flexibility of each sector (Coleman et al., 2020). Capacity and capability can be measured in terms of expanding facilities for routine care, program development (e.g., prevention and treatment programs), staff expertise, global quality standards, and sustainable funding. Multilevel planning for rapid response can be evaluated in terms of the robustness of data systems, management structure and communication systems that support implementation and adaptation, and regional planning for rapid decision making. Specifically, Mansoura noted the importance for regional planning to adapt and change resource deployment, with triggers and systems in place to initiate access to global resources as needed. Health care system competence can be measured in terms of management and staff ability to rapidly change systems and focus, staff training and cross-training (e.g., interactive education programs), and ability to provide online access to educational resources for unanticipated or urgent needs. Finally, global resource access can be measured through assessments of readiness to meet standards, supply chain networks, access to expertise from high-income countries and staff mentorship, and standardized data reporting. Mansoura emphasized the need for readiness assessments to meet standards as a key for global flex competence.

In 2019, the Global Health Security Index was published, measuring the health preparedness of each country.[12] However, the COVID-19 pandemic revealed that this index was not highly effective at predicting countries' pandemic preparedness, and it remains unclear how this can best be measured (Crosby et al., 2020). Still, Mansoura reaffirmed that meaningful measures are required for effective investment.

Challenges and Ways Forward to Leverage Synergies and Build Flex Competence

In moving forward with efforts to leverage synergies and build flex competence, Mansoura highlighted the potential challenge of cultural rifts that can arise as the public health sector mobilizes to address pressing disease outbreaks that may have immense impact on public health, national security, and economic security (Bernard, 2013). She called for the health community

---

[12] More information about the 2019 Global Health Security Index is available at https://www.ghsindex.org (accessed November 7, 2021).

to temper its strongly held convictions and to encourage defense and foreign affairs communities to embrace relevant health issues in the first tiers of policy and budget concerns. However, health professionals and health organizations often have little experience crafting messages and presenting issues in a manner that will sway the critical actors in foreign policy, intelligence, and defense sectors. Mansoura acknowledged that this cannot be blamed solely on public health actors, as the security sector is often unenthusiastic about efforts to prioritize pandemics or other public health issues as security issues. She also noted the importance of building trustful relationships for addressing health issues such as TB, cancer, and COVID-19. The potential consequences of mistrust have recently been demonstrated by the variance in vaccine distribution and vaccination during the COVID-19 pandemic (Cheney, 2021).

Promising findings demonstrate the potential synergistic effect of flex competence, said Mansoura. For example, 940,000 children in contact with TB patients received preventive therapy in 2020, representing a 13 percent increase over 2019 and suggesting that COVID-19 response efforts had a synergistic positive effect on child contact preventive therapy (Global Fund, 2021). Anticipating and preparing for public health crises is the cornerstone of recognizing and leveraging powerful synergies, she added. Resources that are redirected in a crisis response can create major deficits in other health care areas and damage existing structures of care; these consequences can be avoided by preparation and integration efforts across the infectious disease, noncommunicable disease, and preparedness communities.

Environmental Transmission Control Lessons from COVID-19 and Tuberculosis

Presented by Edward Nardell, Harvard Medical School and the T.H. Chan School of Public Health

Nardell described environmental transmission control lessons that can be gleaned from efforts to control TB over many decades and efforts to control COVID-19 since 2020. The COVID-19 pandemic response has benefited from lessons learned through TB control; now, there is ample opportunity to apply lessons from the COVID-19 pandemic to TB control.

Mechanisms of Transmission for Tuberculosis and COVID-19

Nardell compared the mechanisms of transmission that underpin the spread of TB and COVID-19. Although they have much in common, they also have differences that are relevant to determining the most effective means of transmission control. TB is predominantly spread indoors and almost exclusively through airborne transmission and inhaled aerosols because *Mycobacterium tuberculosis* (MTB) must reach the alveolar macrophage to cause infection, which is only possible for particles 1–5 μm in size (Milton, 2020). Furthermore, MTB is environmentally adapted, making it stable in airways and capable of traversing ventilation systems. COVID-19 also spreads mostly indoors through inhaled aerosols. For both TB and COVID-19, large droplet spread and surface spread are relatively less important, and RNA found on surfaces and in air is not replication competent. However, unlike MTB, SARS-CoV-2 has multiple mucosal targets in the eyes, nose, and airways—including angiotensin-converting enzyme receptors in the respiratory tract—making it possible for particles of various sizes (1 μm to greater than 100 μm) to cause infection. SARS-CoV-2 is also unlike MTB in that its envelope RNA viruses are fragile in the environment; no evidence of ventilation duct transmission of SARS-CoV-2 has yet been reported. The infectious dose of MTB can be as low as a single bacterium, while the infectious dose of SARS-CoV-2 is quite high (300–1,000 virus particles). MTB is chronically infectious and mostly spread by symptomatic individuals. In contrast, SARS-CoV-2 can spread asymptomatically for a short infectious period of roughly 48 hours, making it unusual among infectious diseases.

The outbreak of COVID-19 at the Skagit Valley Chorale rehearsal in March 2020 was instrumental in confirming that SARS-CoV-2 is primarily airborne, rather than spread through droplets, said Nardell (Miller et al., 2021).[13] Nardell considered the difference in transmission that is most likely to occur through rebreathed air in an indoor room compared with transmission through the ventilation circuit in a building or other structure. Although a common COVID-19 control recommendation is to improve filters in ventilation systems, SARS-CoV-2 appears to be very delicate and generally incapable of traversing ventilation systems or remaining intact when diluted with air from other rooms. In contrast, Nardell stated, it has been established from a TB outbreak on a naval vessel that TB can readily spread through ventilation systems—if present—and from room to room. At the time of the workshop, COVID-19 is not known to travel through ventilation systems (i.e., infectious viral particles being taken into a ventilation system and then released in a different room to cause infection in the absence of person-to-person contact). Nardell contended that COVID-19 seems to be spread primarily through rebreathed air among persons in the same indoor room, with the implication that changing duct filters—a com-

---

[13] None of the participants who attended the 2.5-hour indoor choir rehearsal were symptomatic, yet 53 of the 61 attendees were later found to have COVID-19 and two attendees died. Strict social distancing and hand sanitization measures were in place, thus large droplet and surface spread are highly unlikely to account for the extent of transmission.

mon recommendation for environmental control of SARS-CoV-2—may not be helpful in reducing transmission.

Air Disinfection for Infectious Disease Control

COVID-19 has raised the profile of air disinfection in poorly ventilated buildings, said Nardell. Because COVID-19 is spread primarily through rebreathed air in indoor rooms, he suggested approaches to air disinfection for COVID-19 control be room-based. Options for room-based air disinfection include natural ventilation, mechanical ventilation, room air cleaners, upper-room germicidal ultraviolet (GUV) air disinfection, and newer technologies brought about by the COVID-19 pandemic.

Natural ventilation—which has been relied upon in TB control for many years—is capable of reducing transmission, but it is highly variable depending on building design and other conditions. Use of natural ventilation for air disinfection is also under threat from the effects of climate change. Mechanical ventilation can help to dilute air and reduce transmission of COVID-19, but this option is rarely available in countries with high TB burdens. Mechanical ventilation is also limited by air flow, thus not an ideal solution. Similarly, room air cleaners have been distributed as a tool for TB control in many countries, but not all models contribute significantly to overall air flow.[14]

Nardell described the benefits of using upper-room GUV for air disinfection. These devices are not limited by air flow; instead, they treat large volumes of air instantaneously, making them highly economical. GUV air disinfection is also safe for room occupants and effective against various infectious disease agents, including MTB, SARS-CoV-2, influenza viruses, and the measles virus. Upper-room GUV air disinfection is an old and affordable technology, but companies have not traditionally been motivated to develop this technology for TB control. However, the COVID-19 pandemic has spurred new developments in upper-room GUV air disinfection that will likely benefit TB control efforts, said Nardell. These advancements include lowered costs, more evidence of efficacy, and expanded support systems for GUV technology. The pandemic has also spurred advancements in ultraviolet technology, he added. New 222-nm "far-UV" devices can be used directly around room occupants without any concern for eye or skin irritation. Although far-UV devices are currently too expensive for widespread use, they will likely become more affordable over time. New ion generators are also being developed in response to the COVID-19 pandemic.

---

[14] Nardell noted that a key concern for measuring air flow is to measure the number of equivalent air changes contributed by a device. Thus, the effectiveness of any ventilation-based disease control is closely linked to the number of equivalent air changes that it provides.

Prevention of COVID-19 and Tuberculosis Transmission Using Upper-Room Germicidal Ultraviolet Systems

Nardell described how upper-room GUV disinfects large volumes of air at one time. In a room with 9-foot ceilings, UV-C radiation is projected throughout the airspace above 7 feet from the ground. This creates a zone of air disinfection in the unoccupied space 2 feet below the ceiling. As contaminated warm air rises, it naturally circulates cooler disinfected air back down into the occupied space. Low-velocity ceiling fans are added to these systems to ensure good air mixing. Unlike upper-room GUV, far UV can be used to disinfect the entire room rather than only unoccupied space.

Use of upper-room GUV has a long history in infectious disease control, said Nardell. A 1942 study demonstrated that upper-room GUV in school rooms effectively prevented the transmission of measles, the most infectious known respiratory pathogen (Wells et al., 1942). Given that measles is far more contagious than COVID-19, upper-room GUV could also stop the spread of COVID-19, which is highly UV-susceptible. Upper-room GUV has also been shown to be 80 percent effective against TB transmission, capable of adding the equivalent of 24 air changes per hour (Mphaphlele et al., 2015).

In addition to being effective in halting transmission, upper-room GUV is also cost-effective, added Nardell. One unpublished study used a renovated hospital room to introduce an aerosolized test organism and perform quantitative air sampling, finding that upper-room GUV was far less expensive per year per equivalent air changes per hour compared to mechanical ventilation or three different commercial air cleaners; in fact, upper-room GUV was more than 9 times more cost-effective than the other technologies (Nardell, 2021).

Effects of Climate Change on Airborne Disease Control

Nardell discussed the effects of climate change on airborne disease control. As temperatures have risen, the use of ductless air conditioning units has expanded. For instance, he found that ductless air conditioning sales in India rose dramatically between 2010 and 2015, and that trend appeared to continue between 2015 and 2021. Because windows are closed when air conditioners are in use and ductless air conditioning units do not use ventilation, ductless air conditioners create unventilated spaces. In addition to cooling spaces, it is also necessary to replace the ventilation lost to ductless air conditioners. This trend is directly linked to increased risk of airborne infection transmission: the risk of airborne infection doubles within 1 hour of closing the windows in a space cooled with ductless air conditioning (Nardell et al., 2020).

Gaps and Opportunities in Management of Latent Tuberculosis Infection

Presented by Gavin Churchyard, the Aurum Institute

Churchyard discussed gaps and opportunities in the management of latent TB infection and barriers to the implementation of TPT. He also identified research gaps within the TB prevention cascade—specifically for people living with TB and HIV and for household contacts of people with TB—and highlighted prospects for future TB regimens. Although progress has been made toward achieving the UN High-Level Meeting targets for 2022 for scaling up the provision of TPT to people of all ages and people living with HIV, efforts to scale up TPT for household contacts have been insufficient to meet the 2022 goals. Notably, less than 1 percent of the targeted 20 million household contacts age 5 years or older have received TPT (WHO, 2020). Churchyard noted that a recent WHO meeting identified barriers to TPT implementation, research gaps along the cascade of prevention, and specific research gaps related to high-risk groups (Oxlade et al., 2021).

Research Priorities in the Implementation of Tuberculosis Preventive Treatment and the Prevention Cascade

At the health system level, barriers to TPT implementation include a lack of priority of TB control programs, limited access to diagnostics and drugs, inadequate financing, and lack of a patient-centered perspective (Oxlade et al., 2021). To overcome those barriers, research priorities include:

- Collecting data to build a stronger public health case for the programmatic management of TPT;
- Creating simplified diagnostic algorithms for TB disease and developing shorter treatment regimens;
- Understanding financing gaps, modeling the cost-effectiveness of TPT, and modeling the effect of TPT on TB incidence and mortality; and
- Better understanding the perspectives of patients and clients in diverse settings about the risks and benefits of TPT.

Research gaps also pervade the cascade of prevention, said Churchyard. He highlighted sets of research needs and priorities in the domains of (1) better identifying and connecting to populations at risk, (2) improving screening and testing for TB infection, (3) more accurately excluding active TB infection, and (4) improving the initiation and completion of TPT (see Box 3-3) (Oxlade et al., 2021).

BOX 3-3
Research Priorities in the Cascade of Tuberculosis Prevention

Identifying and connecting to populations at risk:
1. Evaluate the best approaches for linkage to care.
2. Model the effect of different strategies in different contexts.
3. Explore the acceptability and feasibility of different treatments and models of care.

Improving screening and testing for TB infection:
1. Reevaluate the cost, feasibility, yield, and cost-effectiveness of testing for TB infection among household contacts age 5 years or older.
2. Assess the benefits of testing for TB infection in persons living with HIV who are on antiretroviral therapy and/or in low-burden settings.
3. Evaluate more specific TB skin tests and POC interferon gamma release assay tests.
4. Gain a deeper understanding of the mechanisms of latency to identify biomarkers of TB progression.

More accurately excluding active TB infection:
1. Evaluate the use of computer-aided TB detection via chest X-rays.
2. Assess the cost-effectiveness and feasibility of expanding digital chest X-ray evaluation in primary care settings in high- and intermediate-incidence countries.
3. Estimate the cost-effectiveness of expanding chest X-ray access.
4. Develop and assess alternative models to exclude TB disease other than chest X-ray.

Improving the initiation and completion of tuberculosis preventive therapy (TPT):
1. Evaluate the efficacy, safety, tolerability, and acceptability of 1- to 2-month regimens.
2. Assess patient and provider attitudes to TPT and develop strategies to overcome treatment barriers.
3. Develop accurate methods to monitor and track adverse events related to TPT regimens in programmatic settings.
4. Evaluate the safety of all TPT regimens for pregnant and breastfeeding women.
5. Develop shorter regimens and/or long-acting single-dose regimens.

SOURCES: Adapted from Gavin Churchyard's presentation on September 14, 2021; Oxlade et al., 2021.

Research Progress and Priorities in Tuberculosis Preventive Treatment for High-Risk Groups

Churchyard highlighted research progress and priorities in the provision of TPT to high-risk groups, including people living with HIV, household contacts under 5 years old, household contacts age 5 years or older, and other people at risk.

WHO recommends a range of TPT regimens for people with HIV, including isoniazid and rifapentine for 3 months (3HP) and isoniazid and rifapentine for 1 month (1HP). The DOLPHIN trial showed that 3HP was well tolerated by and safe for people with HIV on antiretroviral therapy without dose adjustment of dolutegravir, and virologic suppression was maintained through the regimen (Dooley et al., 2020). The DOLPHIN TOO trial is amending the original protocol to describe the rate of decline of plasma HIV-1 viral load among antiretroviral naïve participants starting isoniazid preventive therapy or 3HP regimens with a dolutegravir antiretroviral regimen.[15]

TPT guidelines for children younger than 5 are complex, Churchyard explained. Regimens are determined by age, HIV status, and whether or not the antiretroviral therapy includes nevirapine or lopinavir/ritonavir. Consequently, these guidelines require three different child-friendly TPT regimens. The guidelines should be simplified such that all children and older contacts in each household can receive the same TPT regimen, he said. Tuberculosis Trials Consortium Study 35 is a dose-finding and safety study of providing 3HP to HIV-infected and HIV-uninfected children with latent TB infection.[16] The study is testing a child-friendly, fixed-dose combination tablet of 3HP that dissolves in water to optimize doses for the youngest children. In 2022, the DOLPHIN KIDS study will assess the safety, tolerability, and pharmacokinetics of 3 months of 3HP among infants, children, and adolescents living with HIV and taking dolutegravir as an antiretroviral therapy.[17]

The Brief Rifapentine-Isoniazid Evaluation for TB Prevention (BRIEF TB) trial demonstrated the efficacy of an ultrashort course 1HP regimen of daily isoniazid and rifapentine in HIV-positive persons (Swindells et al., 2019).[18] Compared to the 9-month isoniazid regimen, 1HP was noninferior in terms

---

[15] More information about the DOLPHIN TOO trial is available from https://clinicaltrials.gov/ct2/show/NCT03435146 (accessed January 3, 2022).

[16] More information about Tuberculosis Trials Consortium Study 35 is available from https://clinicaltrials.gov/ct2/show/NCT03730181 (accessed December 15, 2021).

[17] More information about the DOLPHIN KIDS study is available from https://clinicaltrials.gov/ct2/show/NCT05122767?term=dolphin+kids&draw=2&rank=1 (accessed January 3, 2022).

[18] More information about Brief Rifapentine-Isoniazid Evaluation for TB Prevention (BRIEF TB) trial is available from https://clinicaltrials.gov/ct2/show/NCT01404312 (accessed December 15, 2021).

of efficacy and superior in terms of safety, tolerability, and treatment completion. Currently, there is no evidence for use of this regimen in HIV-negative persons, children, or pregnant women, and dolutegravir doses may need to be adjusted for HIV-positive patients on antiretroviral therapy.[19] The Impact4TB One-to-Three superiority trial will compare the use of the 1HP regimen to the 3HP regimen in adult and adolescent HIV-positive persons and household contacts in terms of treatment completion, treatment-limiting adverse events, safety, and cost-effectiveness. The study will begin in August 2022 across sites in South Africa, Indonesia, India, and Mozambique.

Churchyard added that more cost-effectiveness data are required to support the increased use of 1HP. The cost-effectiveness of 1HP is driven by 1HP completion rates and efficiency, the cost of rifapentine, and the prevalence of latent TB. The 1HP regimen would cost substantially more to achieve the outcomes currently achieved by 3HP regimens. However, a reduction in the price of rifapentine can significantly lower the regimen cost.

Pregnant women have a higher risk of TB, said Churchyard. Two clinical trials suggest an association between HIV-infected pregnant women receiving isoniazid preventive treatment and increased risk of adverse pregnancy outcomes. Evidence for the use of rifapentine-based TPT regimens among pregnant women is beginning to emerge. The IMPAACT 2001 study provided the first evidence that rifapentine was safe for HIV-infected and HIV-uninfected pregnant women and that the dose of rifapentine need not be adjusted. The WHIP3TB trial has collected data on pregnancy outcomes for pregnant HIV-positive women, which were reported in late 2021 (Chihota et al., 2021). In late 2022, the DOLPHIN MOMS study will evaluate the safety, tolerability, and pharmacokinetics of 1HP in comparison with 3HP initiated antepartum versus postpartum.

Churchyard also discussed the use of TPT for household contacts of TB patients by presenting results from the Protecting Households On Exposure to Newly Diagnosed Index Multidrug-Resistant Tuberculosis Patients (PHOENIx MDR-TB) trial conducted in eight high-burden countries.[20] The PHOENIx MDR-TB feasibility trial demonstrated that 77 percent of household contacts of MDR TB patients were in a high-risk group for developing TB (Gupta et al., 2020). Among household contacts that were not in a risk group at baseline, more than 20 percent tested positive for infection within 1 year, suggesting that the majority of household contacts of MDR TB patients are at risk of developing TB and would benefit from TPT.

---

[19] The A5372 trial will evaluate whether doses of dolutegravir need to be adjusted for patients taking this 1HP regimen.

[20] More information about the Protecting Households on Exposure to Newly Diagnosed Index Multidrug-Resistant Tuberculosis Patients trial is available from https://clinicaltrials.gov/ct2/show/NCT03568383 (accessed December 15, 2021).

However, further research is needed to understand the advantages and disadvantages of testing for TB infection among household contacts. Furthermore, the feasibility trial demonstrated that children younger than 5 years and HIV-infected household contacts age 5 years and older had the greatest risk of developing TB. Research is also needed to understand the epidemiological effects of treating high-risk household contacts of various ages. It has been suggested that TPT has limited value in high-transmission countries because of the risk of reinfection in communities, Churchyard added. One modeling study conducted in 2014 found that while household contact tracing alone may not be sufficient to reduce TB incidence, the combination of TPT with household contact tracing may significantly increase reductions in TB incidence (Kasaie et al., 2014).

To address the gap in evidence from randomized trials on providing TPT for contacts exposed to MDR TB, three trials are underway: the Tuberculosis Child Multidrug-resistant Preventive Therapy trial (TB-CHAMP),[21] the VQUIN MDR trial,[22] and PHOENIx MDR-TB. TB-CHAMP is a cluster randomized, community-based superiority trial providing pediatric dispersible levofloxacin tablets daily for 6 months to children age 5 years or younger. The VQUIN MDR trial is evaluating a 6-month daily levofloxacin regimen in a cluster randomized, community-based superiority trial targeting tuberculin skin test (TST)–positive participants of all ages, including infants less than 6 months old. The PHOENIx MDR-TB trial is comparing 26-week daily regimens of isoniazid or delamanid, targeting children younger than 5, people who are HIV-positive, and people older than 5 who tested positive for TB through either the TST or interferon gamma release assay (IGRA).[23] While awaiting results from these trials, WHO has conditionally recommended the use of a TPT regimen of 6 months daily levofloxacin with or without ethambutol or ethionamide (WHO, 2018).

Future Tuberculosis Preventive Treatment Regimens

Churchyard emphasized the importance of managing the global burden of TB infection to meet End TB targets. In addition to addressing research gaps described above, further research is needed to improve potency and further reduce the duration of treatment for TPT. Although TPT regimens have advanced in recent years, maximizing the benefits of TPT warrants fur-

---

[21] More information about TB-CHAMP is available from https://www.mrcctu.ucl.ac.uk/studies/all-studies/t/tb-champ (accessed December 15, 2021).

[22] More information about the VQUIN MDR trial is available from https://www.woolcockvietnam.org/vquin (accessed December 15, 2021).

[23] There are two tests that can be used to detect TB infection, the tuberculin skin test (or TB skin test, TST) and a blood test to measure release of interferon gamma (IGRA). See https://www.cdc.gov/tb/topic/testing/tbtesttypes.htm (accessed January 3, 2022).

ther innovation, said Churchyard. To that end, additional ultra-short-course regimens are currently being evaluated. The 2R2 trial is comparing the use of higher doses of rifampicin for 2 months with the standard TPT rifampicin dose with the aim of determining whether doubling or tripling the standard dose is safe and effective. The Assessment of the Safety, Tolerability, and Effectiveness of Rifapentine Given Daily for Latent Tuberculosis Infection (ASTERoiD) study is assessing the safety, tolerability, and effectiveness of a 6-week daily rifapentine regimen with regimens between 12 and 16 weeks in length.[24] It may be possible to reduce the duration of TPT for DS TB infections using 2-week regimens containing bedaquiline with rifapentine (Zhang et al., 2011). Furthermore, it may be possible to reduce the duration of TPT for MDR TB contacts to 1 month with bedaquiline alone or in combination with other drugs. Long-acting injectable TB drugs may also hold great promise for TPT in the future, Churchyard added.

---

[24] More information about the ASTERoiD study is available from https://clinicaltrials.gov/ct2/show/NCT03474029 (accessed December 15, 2021).

4

Vaccines and Therapeutics

The second session of the second part of the workshop, which focused on advancements in tuberculosis (TB) vaccines and therapeutics, was moderated by Kent Kester, vice president and head of Translational Science and Biomarkers at Sanofi Pasteur, and Charles Wells, head of Therapeutics Development at the Bill & Melinda Gates Medical Research Institute. The session began with presentations on strategies to make better use of existing tools and new technologies. Alex Schmidt, head of vaccine development at the Bill & Melinda Gates Medical Research Institute, discussed the history and current state of policies regarding the use of the Bacillus Calmette–Guérin (BCG) vaccine and the potential role of BCG revaccination in TB elimination. Steve Reed, cofounder, president, and chief executive officer at HDT Bio, discussed the breadth and diversity of ongoing research in the TB vaccine pipeline. Daniel Kalman, professor of pathology at Emory University School of Medicine, examined the use of host-directed therapeutics for treating antibiotic-resistant TB. Rhea Coler, senior investigator at Seattle Children's Research Institute Center for Global Infectious Disease Research and professor at the University of Washington School of Medicine, focused on immune mechanisms of protection against TB.

The next set of presentations explored strategies to transform treatment options for TB. Payam Nahid, professor of pulmonary and critical care medicine and director of the Center for Tuberculosis at the University of California, San Francisco, described lessons learned from designing and conducting a successful regimen-shortening trial for TB treatment. Adrian Thomas, vice president of Global Strategy, Programs and Policy for Global

Public Health at Johnson and Johnson (J&J), and Norbert Ndjeka, director of drug-resistant TB (DR TB), TB, and HIV at the National Department of Health, South Africa, both discussed the rollout of bedaquiline, a treatment for multidrug-resistant (MDR) TB. David Hermann, deputy director at the Bill & Melinda Gates Foundation Global Health Division overseeing the TB drug initiative, highlighted progress toward a shorter, simpler, safer pan-TB regimen for treating multiple forms of TB. Anna Vassall, director of the London School of Hygiene and Tropical Medicine Global Health Economics Centre and Joep Lang Chair at the Amsterdam Institute for Global Health and Development, discussed the value of conducting context-specific economic analyses of novel TB treatment regimens. The session concluded with reflections on critical elements in the implementation of new treatments for TB. Ezra Tessera, senior advisor of TB surveillance at the TB Data, Impact Assessment, and Communications Hub at U.S. Agency for International Development (USAID), John Snow Institute, focused on patient-centered implications of advancements in TB treatment and care. Richard Chaisson, professor of medicine, epidemiology, and international health and director of the Center for Tuberculosis Research at Johns Hopkins University School of Medicine, emphasized the urgency of framing TB as a global health emergency.

EXISTING TOOLS AND NEW TECHNOLOGIES

Bacillus Calmette–Guérin Revaccination

Presented by Alex Schmidt, Bill & Melinda Gates Medical Research Institute

Schmidt discussed the history and current state of policies regarding the use of the BCG vaccine and whether BCG revaccination can play a role in TB elimination.[1] Over the past century, most countries have implemented national BCG vaccination policies for all individuals (see Figure 4-1).

Evidence for BCG Vaccination

Schmidt noted that because BCG vaccines were first implemented 100 years ago, not all of the evidence supporting the use of BCG meets today's

---

[1] BCG is a vaccine for tuberculosis that consists of live-attenuated *Mycobacterium bovis*, generally found to provide protection from extrapulmonary TB in children. See https://www.cdc.gov/tb/publications/factsheets/prevention/bcg.htm (accessed December 30, 2021).

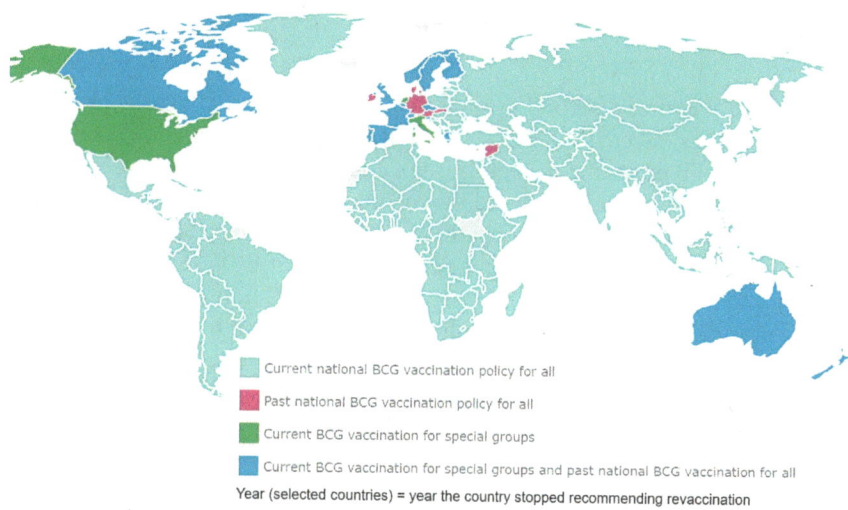

FIGURE 4-1 Bacillus Calmette–Guérin vaccination policies worldwide.
SOURCES: Presented by Alex Schmidt on September 15, 2021; http://www.bcgatlas.org.

evidentiary standards. Furthermore, there have been variations in not only the bacterial strains used in the vaccine, but also variations in geography, incidence, and observed vaccine efficacy. The Ulleval nurses study in Norway, published in 1948, found that BCG was highly efficacious against TB disease, and such studies motivated the introduction of national BCG vaccination policies (Heimbeck, 1948). A large study of adolescents in the UK from 1950 through 1967 who tested negative with a tuberculin skin test found that BCG vaccination was 78.4 percent effective in the prevention of tuberculosis in adolescence and early adulthood (Fourth Report, 1972). Data on the efficacy of BCG vaccines from the United States have been more heterogeneous. A long-term study of BCG in American Indian and Alaska Native communities initiated in 1936 found efficacy rates of around 80 percent in the first 15 years following vaccination and between 50 and 60 percent in subsequent decades, suggesting that primary BCG vaccination protects children and adolescents with negative skin test results from TB (Aronson and Aronson, 1952; Aronson et al., 2004). However, a long-term study of BCG vaccination in children and adults in the southern United States reported only a 14.2 percent BCG vaccination efficacy rate (Comstock and Palmer, 1966). Overall, Schmidt considered, data from children and young adults with negative skin test results who received BCG vaccinations shows that the BCG vaccine provides protection from TB disease.

Evidence for BCG Revaccination

Today, most neonates around the world receive BCG vaccines.[2] Schmidt considered whether a second dose of this vaccine would affect the global TB burden. BCG's vaccine efficacy is known to wane with age and, and since the modern TB epidemic in high-burden countries is mainly driven by cases among adolescents and young adults, neonatal BCG vaccination likely does not continue to offer protection in these older populations. Schmidt discussed two randomized trials that examined the efficacy of BCG revaccination, but also noted that the lack of data regarding baseline TB infection status in the study participants makes these study outcomes difficult to interpret, as BCG is not expected to work in people with current TB infection. One trial in Malawi evaluated a second dose of BCG or BCG plus a killed *Mycobacterium leprae* vaccine in over 23,000 BCG scar-positive children and adults, and found no protective effect for BCG revaccination (Karonga Prevention Trial Group, 1996). The second trial was a cluster randomized trial that studied the effects of BCG revaccination on the incidence of TB in school-age children in Brazil (Barreto et al., 2002, 2011). This study was conducted in two cities and found that revaccination offered no protection in the overall population, but a modest (statistically nonsignificant) effect was observed in Salvador, which is 1,000 km further away from the equator than the second study site in Manaus. One hypothesis to explain this observation is that exposure to environmental mycobacteria, which are more abundant in warmer climates near the equator, may offer protection against TB, therefore diminishing the protective effects of BCG vaccination. Thus, BCG might offer some protection in climates with less abundance of environmental mycobacteria.

A 2018 trial looked at the efficacy of a candidate subunit vaccine H4:IC31 compared with BCG revaccination in preventing *Mycobacterium tuberculosis* (MTB) infection (Nemes et al., 2018). The primary endpoint was prevention of initial interferon gamma release assay (IGRA) conversion, as an indicator of MTB infection, and no statistically significant efficacy was observed. However, evaluation of the secondary endpoint—sustained IGRA conversion defined as an initial conversion that remains positive at 3 and 6 months after the conversion—revealed a 45 percent efficacy for BCG revaccination. While there were fewer initial conversions in the BCG revaccination group compared with the placebo group, the bigger driver of the efficacy read-out was the number of IGRA reversions. He suggested that an optimistic interpretation of this observation is that IGRA reversion—that is,

---

[2] BCG is given as a single dose to neonates in most countries. See https://apps.who.int/immunization_monitoring/globalsummary/schedules?sc%5Br%5D%5B%5D=AFRO&sc%5Br%5D%5B%5D=AMRO&sc%5Br%5D%5B%5D=EMRO&sc%5Br%5D%5B%5D=EURO&sc%5Br%5D%5B%5D=SEARO&sc%5Br%5D%5B%5D=WPRO&sc%5Bd%5D=&sc%5Bv%5D%5B%5D=BCG&sc%5BOK%5D=OK (accessed February 8, 2022).

from having an immune response to MTB proteins to not having an immune response—is indicative that MTB has been cleared, but that cannot yet be conclusively established.

Since no more than 10 percent of latently MTB-infected (IGRA-positive) individuals progress to active TB disease, it is unclear whether a 45 percent reduction in sustained IGRA conversion (prevention of sustained MTB infection) would result in prevention of TB disease. It is possible that a subset of the individuals who reverted to IGRA-negative following BCG revaccination would have never progressed to active disease in the absence of revaccination. Therefore, it is not yet possible to conclude whether the study outcome translates to less development of active TB disease over the longer term, said Schmidt.

An ongoing randomized controlled trial (BCG ReVax) is generating data to potentially support new policies for BCG revaccination.[3] The primary objective of this trial is to demonstrate the efficacy of revaccination in preventing sustained MTB infection, and an important secondary objective is to explore or develop correlates of risk and protection. If the correlates of risk and correlates of protection from the earlier trial can be described and tested in this current large-scale study, it could lead to the identification of candidate indicators for the prevention of sustained MTB infections. This trial will also contribute to an improved understanding of the mechanisms of protection, which is necessary to develop the next generation of vaccines, Schmidt believes. However, it is not clear whether results from this study will be sufficient to spur policy changes such as implementation of BCG revaccination. To convince policy makers to implement BCG revaccination, it may be necessary to draw on additional data sources, including phase 3 trials and real-world evidence from the discontinued BCG revaccination programs.

Current State of Evidence and Ways Forward for BCG Revaccination

Schmidt provided an overview of evidence to date for BCG revaccination and suggested several paths forward to further elucidate the effectiveness of this strategy. BCG revaccination is associated with a higher rate of IGRA reversion. The mechanism of this effect is not yet fully understood, but it could be an indication of a protective immune response that potentially leads to MTB clearance. However, as discussed above, it is unknown what percentage of BCG revaccinated individuals who reverted to IGRA-negative would have progressed to develop TB disease in the absence of IGRA reversion. To demonstrate such a preventive effect, the correlates or indicators

---

[3] This clinical trial was mentioned in Chapter 2. See more information about the NCT04152161 trial at https://clinicaltrials.gov/ct2/show/NCT04152161 (accessed November 18, 2021).

for prevention of sustained infection must be linked to the correlates for prevention of disease.

Given its availability and affordability, BCG revaccination could contribute to accelerating the end of the TB epidemic, but a potential policy change will likely depend on a definitive link between prevention of sustained infection to prevention of disease. The evidence generated by the BCG ReVax study may provide useful data for policy makers considering the implementation of BCG revaccination. Further evidence may be generated by forthcoming randomized controlled trials (e.g., rBCG phase 3)[4] or from real-world data. However, factors such as the potential effects of geography, the abundance of environmental mycobacteria, and differences in commercially available vaccines will likely shape those policy deliberations. Schmidt emphasized that if robust correlates of risk and correlates of protection can be established for TB vaccines, the effect on vaccine development could be transformational, leading to faster, less expensive, and easier-to-iterate vaccines.[5]

Pathway to Effective Tuberculosis Vaccines: Promising New Adjuvants and Late-Stage Clinical Development of Vaccine Candidates

Presented by Steven Reed, University of Washington and HDT Bio

Reed discussed the breadth and diversity of ongoing research in the TB vaccine pipeline within which numerous vaccine candidates are being studied, including those based on live or whole-cell organisms, vector platforms, and recombinant proteins. He explained that there is a range of strategies and potential uses of TB vaccines (see Figure 4-2). For instance, pre-infection vaccines are intended to prevent infection and/or disease by reducing the risk of either the initial infection or establishment of granuloma. Post-infection vaccines aim to prevent disease progression after initial infection and/or prevent reactivation from latent infections. Immunotherapeutic vaccines can be used to treat TB disease, shorten the course of chemotherapy for active TB, and decrease relapse or reinfection rates.

Promising Vaccines and Advancements in Vaccine Technology

Reed suggested that focusing on effective adjuvants for protein vaccines as well as alternative delivery of vaccine antigens, such as delivering antigens via nucleic acids instead of proteins, are two promising research

---

[4] See https://www.clinicaltrials.gov/ct2/show/NCT03152903 (accessed December 30, 2021).

[5] BCG revaccination is a debated topic. For other references related to this topic, see Ahmed et al., 2021.

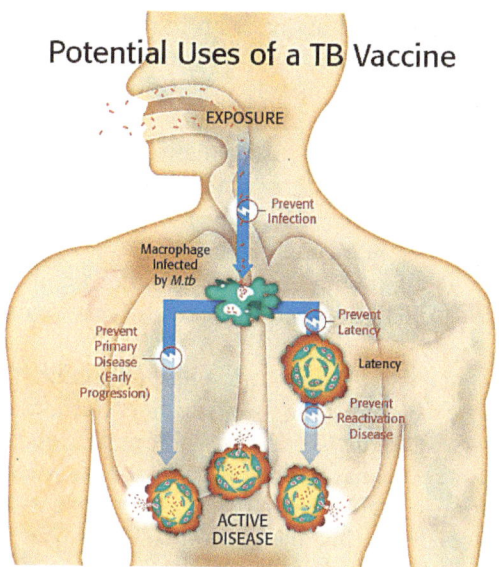

FIGURE 4-2 Potential uses of a tuberculosis vaccine.
NOTE: *M.tb = Mycobacterium tuberculosis.*
SOURCES: Presented by Steve Reed on September 15, 2021; adapted from Bill & Melinda Gates Foundation.

areas to further advance and accelerate TB vaccine development. He shared the example of the M72/AS01$_E$ vaccine, which was developed by Reed and his colleagues over 25 years ago and has been evaluated for its effect in prevention of disease with promising results, but has faced slow progress in advancement since. Reed also discussed potential areas of research that could accelerate the development of promising vaccines, such as M72/AS01$_E$ (Van Der Meeren et al., 2018).[6,7]

Reed highlighted the effect of intellectual property constraints on current toll-like receptor agonists that are used as vaccine adjuvants. In the past, access to several of these components used in adjuvants such as AS01$_E$ has been restricted by intellectual property regulations (e.g., licensing requirements).[8] With the expiration of key patents and the evolution

---

[6] QuantiFERON-TB is an interferon-gamma release assay (IGRA) for the diagnosis of *Mycobacterium tuberculosis* infections. A positive assay result indicates MTB infection. See https://www.cdc.gov/tb/publications/factsheets/testing/igra.htm.

[7] Van Der Meeren et al., 2018, conveys the results of an interim analysis. A final analysis was published by Tait et al., 2019, which demonstrated results of 49.7 percent efficacy.

[8] AS01 stands for Adjuvant System 01 and is a vaccine adjuvant that consists of monophosphoryl lipid A (a TLR4 agonist often derived from bacterial cell membranes) and saponin (a plant-derived natural product) in a liposomal formulation. See Garçon and Di Pasquale, 2017.

of synthetic biology, TLR4 agonists are now freely available and can be derived using synthetic ingredients.[9] Reed explained how synthetic biology may occupy an important role in developing next-generation AS01. AS01 has traditionally been made using natural products, including a semi-synthetic cholesterol that is in high demand for various lipid formulations in pharmaceutical products. Reliance on natural products for production can be expensive. However, synthetic or partially synthetic versions of each of these products are now available, which will broaden access to AS01. Reed encouraged researchers to consider this approach to replicate M72/AS01$_E$ data with a focus on improving global access to vaccination.

New adjuvants also hold great promise in immunotherapy, said Reed. Based on evidence to support the use of vaccines for immune therapy for TB, efforts are underway to further explore this application (Coler et al., 2013). The M72/AS01$_E$ vaccine has been considered for immunotherapy, though its use was discontinued owing to reports of adverse events. Still, Reed posited that one takeaway from this observation could be that the selection of an adjuvant may best be linked to the application, as in whether it is used as part of an immunotherapeutic or as a prophylactic vaccine.

Nucleic Acids as Vaccine Platforms

Reed next discussed nucleic acid vaccine platforms, where instead of using traditional protein antigens, antigen-encoding DNA or RNA is delivered by the vaccine for subsequent transcription or translation to produce the target antigen. He began with RNA vaccines, emphasizing lessons learned from the COVID-19 pandemic. RNA vaccine development has struggled in the past but demonstrated success during the COVID-19 pandemic, building in part on prior research that identified the target protein antigen. However, COVID-19 has also shown that local manufacturing and global access to vaccines are critical for halting pandemics. Accordingly to Reed, RNA vaccines offer numerous important advantages:

- They can be developed using cost-effective synthetic processes.
- They are safe, and they create potent antibody and cellular responses.
- They can also encode multiple antigens, adding to their cost-effectiveness.

Despite the promise of RNA vaccines, the extent and durability of RNA vaccine T-cell responses are not yet known.

---

[9] TLR4 stands for toll-like receptor 4. Toll-like receptors detect pathogens and initiate immune responses. See Celine and Yuanqing, 2014.

In contrast to the recent progress with RNA vaccines, research to develop DNA vaccines has been challenging, Reed said. He believes that DNA vaccines can provide sufficient T-cell response, but methods to effectively deliver DNA immunization (e.g., electroporation) are difficult to achieve. Furthermore, efficient protein expression from DNA vaccination requires the vaccine material to be delivered into the cells' nuclei, while efficient expression of RNA vaccination requires only cytoplasmic delivery. In addition, RNA vaccines may use either nonreplicating mRNA or self-replicating RNA.[10] Reed believes that replicating RNA produces more proteins and generates more virus-like particles, resulting in more potent T-cell responses than mRNA vaccines and requiring smaller doses. Reed noted that his team is focusing on replicating RNA vaccines for these reasons.

Formulation of RNA Vaccines

Lastly, Reed discussed formulation for RNA vaccines. The most common type of formulation has been lipid nanoparticles that encapsulate the RNA. Lipid nanoparticles allow for a single-vial vaccine product, but these products are complex to manufacture and scale up, and each target RNA must be encapsulated within the nanoparticles (Malone et al., 1989). Cationic nanoemulsion RNA vaccine formulations create a kinetic surface chemistry on the oil particles that allows the RNA to adhere to the outside of the particle (Brito et al., 2014). This formulation allows for stockpiling of formulation and rapid use with different target RNAs. However, it also requires a two-vial presentation that can be mixed at bedside. Nanostructured lipid carriers are similar to cationic nanoemulsions, but they include a solid oil component and have historically been used for the delivery of lipophilic small-molecule drugs.

Reed discussed the lipid inorganic nanoparticle (LION) RNA formulation that his team has developed, where adjuvant oils and inorganic metal particles in the core are surrounded by cationic lipids with replicating RNA stabilized on the outside surface. The use of LION or other formulations that have RNA adhered to the outside allows for easier scaling up of production, and the use of replicating RNA could lower the required dose of the potential vaccine. Reed pointed out that these two factors may be critical for TB and COVID-19 control, as controlling these diseases requires a large number of individual doses.

RNA delivery technology has been optimized to provide single shot protection for TB, said Reed. This technology has shown promising results

---

[10] While two nonreplicating, mRNA-based vaccines had received emergency use authorization for COVID-19 at the time of the workshop, self-replicating or self-amplifying RNA vaccines have not yet been approved. See Bloom et al., 2021, for a review on self-replicating or self-amplifying RNA vaccines.

among mice and ideally those results will be predictive of efficacy in non-human primates (NHPs) and humans. Importantly, the delivery of TB protection in a single shot will help meet the need for hundreds of millions of doses of vaccines. HDT Bio has ongoing work to set up centers for technology transfer and capacity development in several countries, including Brazil, South Africa, India, South Korea, and China. Reed added that they have found technology transfer efforts to be very successful in India because of existing efforts conducted by lead investigators in that country.

Advances in Host-Directed Therapeutics for Antibiotic-Resistant Tuberculosis

Presented by Daniel Kalman, Emory University

Kalman discussed how the use of host-directed therapeutics (as opposed to conventional antibiotics) for treating DR TB has the potential to change the development landscape. New solutions are needed to counter both DR TB and TB-induced impairment of lung function, which is associated with a substantial global economic burden (Menzies et al., 2021). Host-directed therapeutics for TB may help address both of those issues by circumventing antibiotic resistance and improving lung function.

Kalman suggested that COVID-19 may increase deaths from bacterial infections by causing impaired antibacterial immune responses—a condition that Kalman classified as "immune amnesia."[11] Kalman worried that COVID-19-induced lymphopenia may have similar consequences, further surmising that COVID-19 patients with lung damage may be more susceptible to TB and vice versa. Moreover, COVID-19 pandemic response measures have led to reductions in TB control in Africa. Given these challenges, he considered whether host-directed therapeutics may offer a solution.

Development of the Host-Directed Therapeutic Imatinib

Host-directed therapeutics were originally developed for malaria, Kalman noted. They offer activity against antibiotic-resistant strains because they target the host, reducing the likelihood of developing antibiotic resistance, and it is possible for host-directed therapeutics to synergize with

---

[11] Immune amnesia is a term applied to the loss of immune memory described after infection by the measles virus. See Gorvett, 2021. Influenza is also associated with subsequent susceptibility to bacterial lung infections owing to immunological mechanisms; see Paget and Trottein, 2019.

antibiotics. Furthermore, host-directed therapeutics may act against non-replicating MTB.[12]

Kalman discussed an example of host-directed therapeutics with imatinib, a tyrosine kinase inhibitor that is approved for cancer and certain types of blood disorders (brand name: Gleevec).[13] He shared that the development process began with three research questions: (1) how do pathogens move into, throughout, and out of host cells; (2) how can the host immune response be altered to disrupt pathogen–host equilibrium in chronic infections; and (3) is it possible to target immune or cellular functions that MTB has evolved to circumvent? Kalman focused on the ABL1 gene, which appears to mediate the trafficking of MTB within cells by preventing lysosomal fusion, allowing TB to stay outside of the lysosome (Korbee et al., 2018).

Use of Imatinib to Treat Tuberculosis

Kalman explained that in addition to being safe and effective as a chemotherapeutic agent, imatinib is also effective in "resetting" the immune response to TB through stimulating emergency hematopoiesis and has shown promise of potentiating the efficacy of existing antibiotics against MTB (Napier et al., 2011, 2015).[14] Evidence supporting the use of imatinib have been generated in primate infection models. Treatment with imatinib in NHPs with active TB infection was found to increase myelopoiesis. Kalman described a model wherein active or latent TB infection was established in rhesus macaques. In this model, latent TB can be reactivated by additional infection with simian immunodeficiency virus. The animals with active TB were treated at the peak of disease with either imatinib and antibiotics or with antibiotics alone. NHPs with reactivated latent TB were treated with imatinib alone (no antibiotics). Survival rates among these NHPs are lowest among those with active TB, but the combination of imatinib with antibiotics was found to reduce bacterial load more than antibiotics alone. With reactivated TB, imatinib was also found to reduce bacterial load. This finding suggested that using imatinib may be useful for reducing the length of treatment. Furthermore, chest X-ray imaging showed that imatinib reduced signs of pulmonary disease in TB-infected animals. Kalman added that imatinib was also shown to reduce disease pathology by reducing granulomas,

---

[12] Nonreplicating or dormant *M. tuberculosis* in the patient are recalcitrant to treatment with typical antibiotics treatment. See Connolly et al., 2007.

[13] Kalman noted that imatinib was initially developed for chronic myelogenous leukemia. One of its targets is ABL1 (also known as c-ABL).

[14] Emergency hematopoiesis is a process where hematopoietic stem cells are activated to differentiate and generate immune cells in response to stress signals, including bacterial infections. See Zaretsky et al., 2014.

which may contribute to the observation of synergy between imatinib and antibiotics.

Ongoing Imatinib Dosing Trials

IMPAc-TB has begun a phase 2 trial in collaboration with the National Institutes of Health (NIH) to find the right dose of imatinib, said Kalman.[15] The trial will investigate the safety, pharmacokinetics, and hematologic effects of low doses of imatinib in healthy volunteers when it is given with and without isoniazid and rifabutin. This trial will test the hypothesis that imatinib increases myelopoiesis at low doses and promotes MTB killing ex vivo. Another phase 2 trial will compare the combination of imatinib and antibiotics against the use of antibiotics alone in adult patients with drug-susceptible (DS) TB. This trial will test the hypothesis that imatinib shortens treatment period (measured as a decrease in the time needed to achieve negative sputum culture) and improves lung function.

Prospects for Imatinib Regulatory Approval and Clearance for Use

Kalman discussed regulatory progress toward approval and clearance for imatinib use in TB patients by 2025.[16] Dosing and safety trials in normal patients are underway and expected to be complete by the end of 2022. Efficacy trials are being developed, and an efficacy trial for TB patients with the Aurum Institute in South Africa is in progress. In the future, it will be necessary to test the use of imatinib in patients with MDR TB, he noted. Because imatinib is off-patent (i.e., cheaper generics may be available if there is sufficient market demand) and its safety is well established (thus reducing the need for further expensive clinical trials), the use of imatinib to treat TB is commercially viable. To deliver imatinib as a TB treatment globally, a commercialization and distribution plan will be needed for high-burden countries such as Africa, China, India, and Russia. Currently, imatinib is relatively expensive, but Kalman predicted that as it becomes widely used for TB treatment, the price will drop rapidly. He suggested that the distribution and sale of imatinib for TB treatment could eventually use a commercial

---

[15] The Immune Mechanisms of Protection against *Mycobacterium tuberculosis* Centers (IMPAc-TB) program is an initiative established by the National Institute of Allergy and Infectious Diseases. See https://www.niaid.nih.gov/research/immune-mechanisms-protection-mycobacterium-tuberculosis (accessed December 31, 2021).

[16] At the time of this publication, imatinab was one potential host-directed therapeutic candidate for TB among many others. For a landscape review of host-directed therapeutics, see Young et al., 2020.

model wherein a slimmer profit margin from low pricing is offset by the high volume of doses.

Immune Mechanisms of Protection Against Tuberculosis

Presented by Rhea Coler, Seattle Children's Research Institute

Coler focused on immune mechanisms of protection against TB by providing an overview of the immunology of MTB infection, possible targets of vaccine development, innate and adaptive (mucosal and humoral) immune systems, and correlates of protection. She also introduced work that she and her colleagues are conducting related to the IMPAc-TB study.

Coler pointed out that it has been more than two decades since the World Health Organization (WHO) first declared TB to be a global health emergency and emphasized both the burden of TB and the need to develop new products to prevent, diagnose, and cure the disease. However, progress toward these aims has been slow. In 2020, approximately 10 million people developed TB and 1.4 million people died of the disease. The spread of TB is influenced by a variety of factors, including age, geography, socioeconomic status, and comorbidities. Furthermore, it is known that DR TB is a major contributor to the burden of antimicrobial resistance, which itself is a significant threat to global health security. Each of these factors has implications for strategies for disease control.

Immune Response to Mycobacterium Tuberculosis

Many immune mechanisms have been proposed to control TB, including innate immune responses, antibodies, innate cell interactions by Fc receptors, and lung-resident T cells. Coler described the respiratory mucosal responses following MTB infection of airway epithelial cells (Brazier and McShane, 2020; Stylianou et al., 2019). MTB enters the body via aerosolized droplets that are inhaled into the airways. Although alveolar macrophages are the principal target of these bacilli, they are also capable of infecting human lung epithelial cells. These airway epithelial cells express a variety of pattern recognition receptors. Further, there are surfactant proteins that combine with components of the mycobacterial cell wall. The epithelial recognition of MTB activates numerous signaling pathways that induce the production of cytokines, such as tumor necrosis factor alpha, interferon gamma, and chemokines, such as interleukin (IL)-6 and IL-8. These airway epithelial cells are also potent responders to cytokines, such as IL-1 beta and type 1 interferons released by infected macrophages. Epithelial cells are capable of directly presenting intracellular antigens to resident CD8 T cells through major histocompatibility complex class I molecules, which stimulate interferon gamma production.

Technical Feasibility of Vaccine Development

Several factors support the technical feasibility of a vaccine, said Coler. For instance, it is estimated that 90 percent of persons infected with MTB do not progress to active disease.[17] Additionally, the history of the BCG vaccine supports the feasibility of a vaccine for TB. However, the BCG vaccine is only partially protective in children and prevents only 5 percent of vaccine-preventable deaths attributable to TB, underscoring the need for an alternative vaccine. Moreover, because the term *tuberculosis* is used to refer to multiple diseases,[18] a variety of vaccines may be needed to prevent infection, prevent disease progression, or be used as treatment or adjunctive immunotherapy.

Coler explained that a principal barrier to MTB vaccine development is the complexity of the immune response to infection, along with uncertainty regarding what constitutes immunological correlates of protection. NIH has awarded three contracts to IMPAc-TB with the aim of comprehensively identifying the complex immune responses required to prevent MTB infection or active disease by comparing and investigating the mycobacteria- and vaccine-induced protective immunity in animal and human subjects. IMPAc-TB is working with its partner investigators to advance understanding of the basic immunological mechanisms that regulate host resistance to MTB and vaccine-mediated protection. The hope is that this work will lead to new insights into TB vaccination, she added.

Roadblocks to Vaccine Development

Coler discussed known roadblocks to vaccine development, approaches to overcoming these obstacles, and how the results of those efforts would facilitate effective vaccine development. The current lack of immune correlates has limited the development of vaccine candidates with clinical efficacy. This barrier may be overcome through specific and exploratory immune system interrogation of local (i.e., mucosal) and systemic responses across multiple interventions in preclinical and clinical models, combined with statistical analysis of immune responses. The resulting correlates of protection would help to accelerate the vaccine development pipeline and facilitate a

---

[17] Progression to active TB is host dependent and is affected by factors such as host age. See Narasimhan et al., 2013.
[18] Different forms of TB include active disease, latent infection, and extrapulmonary TB. See https://tbfacts.org/types-of-tb (accessed December 31, 2021).

more rational vaccine design process.[19] However, the tool sets available for high-throughput standardized vaccine candidate evaluation are currently limited. This barrier can be approached by aligning mycobacterial and vaccine intervention regimens and kinetics of host immune interrogation across mouse, guinea pig, NHP, and human studies. Such efforts would facilitate vaccine development through model alignment; furthermore, standardization could be used to test novel candidates with greater throughput.

The effect of prior nontuberculous mycobacteria (NTM) infection on vaccine efficacy also presents challenges to vaccine development, said Coler. These challenges can be approached through evaluation of vaccine efficacy and concurrent immune response while accounting for NTM exposure (preclinical) or positive NTM recall responses (clinical). This approach will support the rational design of TB-specific vaccines that preclude NTM interference and improve efficacy, further informing clinical trial participant criteria. Uncertainty regarding the effect of prior BCG interventions on vaccine efficacy is another challenge for vaccine development. This can be addressed through the evaluation of vaccine efficacy and concurrent immune responses while accounting for planned BCG exposure (preclinical) or positive BCG recall response (clinical). This approach will facilitate the development of rationally designed TB-specific vaccines to preclude BCG vaccine interference or strengthen and enhance BCG vaccination. Finally, the narrow focus on single-vaccine platforms in head-to-head comparison is a barrier to vaccine development. She suggested that this barrier can be approached through specific and exploratory immune system interrogation across multiple interventions. BCG priming, protein antigen and adjuvant combinations, and RNA vaccine candidates can each be explored. This will allow for the design of TB-specific vaccines that positively influence lung pathology and offer protective efficacy with long-lasting immune responses. This approach will also inform platform development decisions so platforms can meet correlates of protection requirements.

Immune Mechanisms of Protection Against Mycobacterium tuberculosis *Center Program*

Coler presented an overview of the IMPAc-TB program, which is a cross-species mechanistic interrogation of mycobacterial and vaccine-induced immunity. The overarching paradigm of IMPAc-TB is to identify and validate common protective correlates of immunity against MTB in

---

[19] Rational vaccine design is an approach where antigens, adjuvants, and delivery systems are combined to elicit an expected immune response against the target pathogen. This is distinct from the historically used empirical vaccine design approach. See Rueckert and Guzmán, 2012.

order to escalate preclinical animal models of TB, NTM exposure, and human challenge experimental medicine studies. She posited that these efforts will be critical for the rational designing and development of candidate vaccines that generate robust levels of durable, protective immunity against TB. The program is using three animal models and human hosts, and it will harmonize assays across various partner sites. The program will use state-of-the-art technologies to increase vaccine efficacy, optimize vaccine delivery, and dissect the immune responses dictated by candidate vaccines. The aim is that novel vaccine candidates can be tested and used with greater throughput through harmonization strategies, such as clinical grading of different BCG vaccines, ultra-low-dose models, various clinical MTB isolates, and various immunological stimulation reagents, such as the MTB 300 peptide pools and NTM peptide pools.

Coler highlighted three contracts that IMPAc-TB was awarded in 2019. Two of these contracts are located at Seattle Children's Research Institute and the University of Washington. Given the close proximity of these facilities, collaboration and synergies are expected to be amplified. The third grant was awarded at the Harvard T.H. Chan School of Public Health. The IMPAc-TB program will use cutting-edge technologies to better understand the immune responses that provide protection against TB infection. She highlighted collaborative efforts within the IMPAc-TB program. Program participants use shared controls, serum samples, and barcoded MTB strains for competition assays, allowing for plug-and-play compatibility between sites. The program also shares standard operating procedures and protocols. She noted that the program organizers hope to back-translate human results into experimental models so they can be more rapidly advanced.[20]

TRANSFORMING TREATMENT OPTIONS

Developing a New Treatment-Shortening Regimen for Drug-Susceptible Tuberculosis

Presented by Payam Nahid, University of California, San Francisco

Nahid described lessons learned from designing and conducting a trial that was successful in developing a new shorter regimen to advance TB treatment to serve as a potential blueprint for future treatment-shortening work. The Tuberculosis Trials Consortium Study 31/AIDS Clinical Trials Group

---

[20] Back-translating refers to incorporation of new knowledge from the disease in humans to inform the improvement of existing or development of new animal models. See Denayer et al., 2014.

A5349 (TBTC Study 31/A5349) was a randomized, open-label, phase 3, noninferiority trial that was co-funded by the Centers for Disease Control and Prevention (CDC) Tuberculosis Trials Consortium and the NIH AIDS Clinical Trials Group (Dorman et al., 2021).[21] This international multicenter study spanned 34 sites in 13 countries across 4 continents.

Study Design and Conduct

TBTC Study 31/A5349 was a three-arm trial that compared two investigational 4-month rifapentine-based regimens with a standard 6-month control regimen. More than 2,500 participants (age 12 years or older) newly diagnosed with DS pulmonary TB were enrolled in the study.[22] The primary efficacy outcome was survival free of tuberculosis at 12 months post-randomization.

The 6-month control arm regimen, endorsed by the CDC and WHO, included 8 weeks of once-daily isoniazid, rifampicin, pyrazinamide, and ethambutol (2HRZE) and followed by 18 weeks of once-daily isoniazid plus rifampicin (4HR). Both investigational arms substituted dose-optimized rifapentine for rifampicin. Participants in the rifapentine-only investigational arm were treated with a regimen of 8 weeks of once-daily isoniazid, rifapentine, pyrazinamide, and ethambutol (2HPZE) followed by 9 weeks of once-daily isoniazid and rifapentine (2HP). Participants in the other investigational arm, which substituted moxifloxacin for ethambutol, received a regimen of once-daily rifapentine, isoniazid, pyrazinamide, and moxifloxacin for 8 weeks followed by once-daily rifapentine, isoniazid, and moxifloxacin for 9 weeks (2HPM). Rifapentine was administered at a dose of 1,200 mg daily—based on extensive pharmacometric modeling work—and moxifloxacin administered at 400 mg daily in accordance with the package insert; the other drugs were given at standard body-weight-adjusted doses. Five of the seven daily doses per week were administered via directly observed treatment. Rifapentine was given with food and rifampicin without, because of the differential food effect on the two drugs.

Efficacy Results and Safety Outcomes

The results of the study demonstrate that the 2HPZM/2HPM regimen is safe and effective for treating DS TB, said Nahid. He presented the pri-

---

[21] This clinical trial was mentioned in Chapter 2. More information about the Tuberculosis Trials Consortium Study 31/AIDS Clinical Trials Group A5349 is available from https://clinicaltrials.gov/ct2/show/NCT02410772 (accessed December 15, 2021).

[22] Participants with HIV co-infection were included with a CD4 threshold of ≥100 cells/mm^3.

mary efficacy results of the study, which had a noninferiority design with a margin of 6.6 percent (see Figure 4-3). To demonstrate noninferiority, the upper bound of the 95 percent confidence interval for the difference in proportions of unfavorable outcomes between investigational and control regimen had to be below 6.6 percent. Noninferiority also had to be demonstrated in both the assessable population and microbiologically eligible study populations.[23]

Compared to the control regimen, the rifapentine-moxifloxacin regimen met the noninferiority criteria for efficacy for both of the co-primary analysis populations, with the upper bound of the 95 percent confidence interval well within the margin across all analyses. The rifapentine-only arm did not meet noninferiority criteria for efficacy versus the control arm in either co-primary analysis population. Nahid added that the results of 14 pre-specified sensitivity analyses, as well as pre-specified analyses conducted in the intention to treat per protocol, were all consistent in meeting noninferiority for this new experimental 17-week rifapentine-moxifloxacin regimen; the rifapentine-only regimen did not meet the noninferiority criteria throughout those analyses.

The primary safety outcome—experiencing any grade 3–5 adverse event during study treatment—was comparable across the three study arms, experienced by 19.3 percent of participants in the control arm,

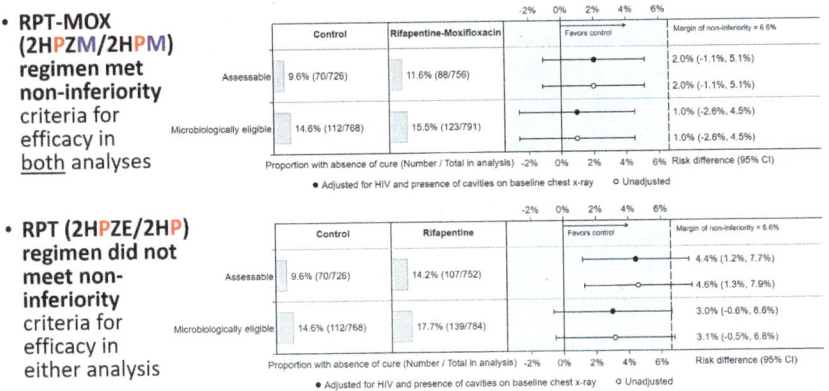

FIGURE 4-3 Primary efficacy results for Tuberculosis Trials Consortium Study 31/ AIDS Clinical Trials Group A5349.
NOTES: CI = confidence interval. Abbreviations for the individual drugs in the treatment regimen are color-coded.
SOURCE: Presented by Payam Nahid on September 15, 2021.

---

[23] More information on the study analysis and criteria are described in Dorman et al., 2021.

14.3 percent of participants in the rifapentine-only arm, and 18.8 percent of participants in the rifapentine-moxifloxacin arm. In secondary safety analyses, there were some numerical but not statistically significant differences across the study arms. Participants in the rifapentine-moxifloxacin arm had a slightly higher proportion of treatment-related grade 3–5 events compared to the control arm. This could be attributed to the open-label trial design because treatment relatedness of the reported adverse events was determined by site investigators unblinded to the regimen. The proportions of participants with treatment discontinuations, at least one serious adverse event during study treatment, and all-cause death during study treatment were slightly lower in participants on both rifapentine regimens compared to the control.

Comparative Context for the New Regimen

Nahid situated the results of this safe and effective 4-month 2HPZM/2HPM regimen within the context of other recent randomized controlled trials for DS TB treatments among microbiologically eligible analysis populations. The rifapentine-moxifloxacin regimen in TBTC Study 31/A5349 is the most potent regimen study to date and is the only regimen that has met noninferiority criteria for efficacy. Although the rifapentine-only regimen in TBTC Study 31/A5349 did not meet noninferiority criteria, it is still the second-most potent regimen compared to other recent trials of treatment-shortening regimens, including: (1) isoniazid-rifampicin-pyrazinamide-moxifloxacin/isoniazid-rifampicin-moxifloxacin (REMoxTB, 2014),[24] (2) moxifloxacin-rifampicin-pyrazinamide-ethambutol/moxifloxacin-rifapentine (RIFAQUIN, 2013), (3) moxifloxacin-rifampicin-pyrazinamide-ethambutol/moxifloxacin-rifampicin (REMoxTB, 2014), and (4) pretomanide-moxifloxacin-pyrazinamide (TB Alliance, 2022).

Advancing Treatment Regimen Development Through Lessons from Previous Studies

Nahid explained that the study design for this safe and effective 4-month 2HPZM/2HPM regimen was informed by lessons from more than two decades of murine, preclinical, and pharmacokinetic studies around rifapentine, which was initially used intermittently. Pharmacometric studies then established animal and human linkages and integrated that knowledge in terms of the effectiveness and efficacy of the rifapentine regimens.

---

[24] More information about REMoxTB, is available from https://www.tballiance.org/portfolio/trial/5093 (accessed December 15, 2021).

This foundational information effectively reduced the risk of many of the study design decisions for TBTC Study 31/A5349. For instance, the study consortium prioritized experimental murine models throughout and conducted iterative phase 2 trials with moxifloxacin-rifapentine. Further, it embedded intensive, sparse, and specific pharmacokinetic substudies to support exposure-response analysis. This allowed for extensive modeling of pharmacokinetic efficacy data, tolerability data, and biomarker data to define the effect of key variables (e.g., sex, race, cohabitation status, HIV status, food effect) in determining the optimal dose. Nahid noted that contrary to prior development approaches, the investigators did not seek to establish the lowest effective dose or the maximally intermittent dose. Rather, they targeted the dose that would facilitate the maximum tolerated exposure, representing a change in the perspective on regimen development for DS TB.

Quantitative Translation Toolbox for Tuberculosis Regimen Development

A quantitative translational toolbox is now available for TB regimen development that is spurring advancement in the field (Ernest et al., 2021). This toolbox integrates multifaceted sources of data on the preclinical side, including plasma pharmacokinetics, lesion pharmacokinetics, immunology, pharmacokinetics/pharmacodynamics of monotherapies, multitherapies, and drug resistance. Also on the preclinical side, new biomarkers—such as the ribosomal RNA (rRNA) synthesis ratio[25]—are providing orthogonal information far beyond that provided by the traditional marker, colony-forming units (Walter et al., 2021). Nahid added that on the clinical side, there is emerging value in looking across lesion pharmacokinetics and then integrating data and information from phase 2A studies and beyond, beginning a new chapter in TB regimen development.

Mitigating Risk Through Study Design and Conduct

The investigators were also able to mitigate risk and optimize lessons from Study31/A5349 through the design and conduct of the trial itself, said Nahid. The large sample size (more than 2,500 participants) allowed for assessment across subgroups, which was useful given the uncertainty at the outset as to whether the regimen would be effective against TB disease of various degrees of cavitary severity. By embedding sparse pharmacokinetics in the study protocol across all arms for all TB drugs and participants, the

---

[25] The rRNA synthesis ratio measures the effect of drugs on ongoing bacterial rRNA synthesis.

trial provides the richest data set available to date with broad geographic representation, including information about the standard 6-month control regimen in addition to the new regimen. Thus, the data set can serve as a benchmark for future TB regimen development work. Owing to uncertainties related to the potential for drug–drug interactions between efavirenz and high-dose rifapentine, enrollment of HIV-positive participants was staged with pharmacokinetics and viral load assessments to assess safety; the two drugs were found to be safely co-administered. The trial also focused upon measuring adherence and maximizing retention; both must be robust to provide practical understanding of how regimens perform in the field—a concept referred to as "high assay sensitivity for noninferiority" by regulatory authorities.

Additionally, the study investigators invested in a multiyear, multinetwork effort to harmonize laboratory practices across sites, based on decades of mycobacteriology experiences, to help reduce noise and differences in data readout across sites (Dorman et al., 2020). Despite these standardized practices often differing from local practices, they were adopted uniformly at the study sites around the world, said Nahid. Real-time data management and reports facilitated quality assurance at sites as well as supporting monitoring and reviews by the Data Safety Monitoring Board. Moreover, the investigators prioritized efforts to minimize bias when measuring endpoints in this open-label study by providing extensive trainings on the trial's standard operating procedure and by developing a new "Possible Poor Treatment Response" procedure.[26] The latter is a guide to collecting a standardized suite of data to understand patient-specific endpoints when investigators are concerned about trial participants. They also embedded substudies of innovative biomarkers, pharmacokinetics, and other investigations co-funded by NIH and others (e.g., intensive pharmacokinetics analyses from this data pool, TBTC Study 31A and 31B to analyze sputum transcriptomics, quantitative GeneXpert indications of treatment outcome, and bacterial drug susceptibility) to learn more from the trial even if the regimen had not proven to be safe and effective. Nahid concluded by highlighting major lessons learned during the design and conduct of Study31/A5349 (see Box 4-1). Additional relevant lessons from the design and conduct of recent TB therapeutics trials are also summarized in a special collection "Advances in Clinical Trial Design for Development of New Treatments for Tuberculosis" (Lienhardt and Nahid, 2019).

---

[26] Nahid noted at the time of the workshop that the manuscript for the "Possible Poor Treatment Response" procedure is under development.

> **BOX 4-1**
> **Overview of Lessons Learned from TBTC Study 31/A5349**
>
> 1. Build upon past work in TB regimen development and be aware of shortcuts that can undermine success.
> 2. Include experimental models—such as murine studies, novel biomarkers, and new tools—as nonnegotiable components of TB treatment regimen development.
> 3. Prioritize preclinical work using new tools that provide orthogonal information.
> 4. Test exact regimens, and interpret the results cautiously.
> 5. Establish appropriate phase 2 study designs—including PK/PD studies of biomarkers—at the outset to de-risk decisions.
> 6. Build in protections to avoid "putting all your eggs in one basket."
> 7. Add substudies to learn more.
> 8. Combine broad, representative recruitment with program-based studies to maximize lessons from real-world experience and aid in the adoption of global policies regarding regimens for treating DS TB (e.g., WHO recently endorsed 4-month once-daily rifapentine, isoniazid, pyrazinamide, and moxifloxacin for 8 weeks followed by once-daily rifapentine, isoniazid, and moxifloxacin for 9 weeks. as an acceptable regimen).
> 9. Engage in robust, effective collaboration to build trust and facilitate the effective study completion.
>
> SOURCE: Adapted from Payam Nahid presentation, September 15, 2021.

Rolling Out a New Treatment Regimen for Drug-Resistant Tuberculosis: Industry Perspective

Presented by Adrian Thomas, Johnson & Johnson

Thomas presented a case study of the rollout of bedaquiline, a treatment for MDR TB. This drug led to the founding of the Global Public Health team at J&J, which addresses HIV, TB, mental health, soil-transmitted helminths, global surgery, a vaccines portfolio, and an early development portfolio that includes dengue fever, malaria, and postpartum hemorrhage. The group uses a model of collaboration at scale, working with over 100 partners at the global, regional, and local levels. The Global Public Health team has its own research and development (R&D) organization, a fully dedicated and accessible team, and an implementation team that works in 26 countries. Using expertise in insight generation, consumer marketing, and human-centered design, the team brings broad business skills and capabilities to the areas it serves.

J&J's Tuberculosis Initiatives

Thomas noted that J&J has long been committed to addressing TB, particularly DR TB. In December 2012, bedaquiline—the first novel mechanism of action TB drug released in nearly 50 years—was approved. Phase 2 data indicated potential for QT interval prolongation[27] and cardiotoxicity. Given the settings within which J&J implements new technologies, creating the infrastructure to monitor for these conditions using electrocardiogram (ECG) and other technology was a challenge. Additionally, reticence to adopt new technologies created an adoption curve for TB that looks very different than for commercial therapeutic areas such as oncology or immunology. Thomas described that, to date, J&J has shipped over 420,000 6-month treatments to MDR TB patients in 147 countries, 47 of which have formal regulatory approvals in place.

A 10-year J&J initiative, spanning from 2018 to 2028, aims to broaden access to TB treatment, improve detection of undiagnosed cases, and accelerate R&D to discover next-generation treatments. An innovation toward expanded access came in the form of a regulatory waiver issued by WHO, which enabled the rapid increase and adoption of treatment in some of the most difficult countries to expand access. For instance, the Democratic Republic of the Congo can have a time lag of 8–12 years for innovation to reach full regulatory approval or adoption. Thomas emphasized the role of USAID, the Stop TB Partnership's Global Drug Facility, WHO, and the Global Fund in supporting the donation program with flexibility, amplifying medical education for appropriate use, and building the infrastructure for ECG monitoring and resistance testing. Private-sector constituency partnerships have also played a large role in expanding access for TB treatment and diagnostic capability. One such partnership is with Cepheid, the company that manufactures the GeneXpert platform used in diagnosing MDR TB and determining the drug resistance profiles. Cepheid and J&J worked with the Chinese government to conduct a pilot TB case-finding study that covered 10 million persons in western provinces of China. The study found the prevalence of DR TB in that region to be about twice the country's previous estimate and created a novel and accelerated pathway to care in China that has continued during the COVID-19 pandemic, said Thomas.

Partnerships and collaboration are also important to research efforts, Thomas noted. Since beginning the 10-year TB initiative in 2018, J&J has continued to progress in the development of bedaquiline, producing a pediatric

---

[27] QT interval prolongation is a heartbeat irregularity in which the Q and T waves, during which heart cells repolarize after a contraction, are longer than normal. See Al-Khatib et al., 2003.

formulation and completing pediatric trials.[28] J&J has advanced an early portfolio in discovery and early science, as well as pursuing licensing partnerships with other private-sector entities. He described how private-sector companies across the pharmaceutical and diagnostic industries have formed partnerships with one another in addition to collaborating with academic, government, and nonprofit organizations. For example, in 2021, J&J launched the Satellite Center for Global Health Discovery at the London School of Hygiene and Tropical Medicine. The Project to Accelerate New Treatments for Tuberculosis (PAN-TB) was established with a consortium of philanthropic, nonprofit, private-sector, and academic partners. Additionally, J&J has joined the Innovative Medicines Initiative to develop new TB antibiotics in collaboration with eight European and academic biotechnology partners.

Collaboration to Address the Challenge of Tuberculosis in South Africa

Thomas described the work J&J has carried out in conjunction with the government of South Africa, USAID, local implementing partners, nongovernmental organizations (NGOs), academic institutions, and health delivery services to comprehensively address the challenge of TB in South Africa. This effort required the creation of a novel paradigm for innovation delivery in the pharmaceutical industry. Typically, new technologies are rapidly absorbed into health systems and followed by cycles of innovation. However, in this case, the delivery model first needed to be broken down to address six different areas: access, medical education, appropriate use, data generation, patient finding, and awareness campaigns. Increasing access involved expanding regulatory access, establishing a donation program to fuel familiarity and use, and aggressive equity-based tiered pricing to ensure affordability and sustainability. Medical education was important in communicating the need for monitoring for QT prolongation with bedaquiline and audiometry testing for signs of early ototoxicity of injectable aminoglycosides, said Thomas. This was seen when South Africa led the world in the move to all-oral, noninjectable regimens for DR TB. Appropriate use refers to ensuring that the appropriate diagnostic technologies are used for DR TB patients and that patients remain on therapy to avoid early development of resistance. It also involves investment in background surveillance programs to monitor for the emergence of drug resistance in the prevalent population.

Thomas stated that data generation has been key, and that South Africa led the effort of establishing the world's largest cohort analysis of DR TB patients. This analysis occurred twice over 5 years and showed that the survival rate for patients with XDR TB increased from 20 percent to 80 percent, resulting in a series of guideline changes, both at WHO and at the local ministry level. This illustrated the dynamic effect the introduction of

---

[28] See https://clinicaltrials.gov/ct2/show/NCT02354014 (accessed December 31, 2021).

a new technology can have. Lastly, awareness campaigns about TB disease and the availability of less-toxic treatments that provided faster sterilization, faster cures, and better overall survival have been critically important, Thomas noted. Mass media and social media were used for above-the-brand communication starting in 2012 and are continuing today.

Lessons Learned in Collaborating Toward a TB-Free South Africa

Thomas emphasized that these efforts required collaboration at every level. Global, catalytic, capacity-building partnerships worked to understand how to best use resources and contribute capabilities, technologies, and products with organizations such as USAID. Global networks allowed implementing partners to bring innovation to the people who need it. Stop TB Partnership's Global Drug Facility created a unique 188-pill bottle that contains a complete course of therapy with simplified regulatory language in four languages. This design enabled therapy availability in 140 countries through a regulatory waiver and a regulatory approval mechanism that accelerated access to patients. Additionally, the Global Drug Facility established an agreement to rapidly decrease the lowest pricing tier to ensure access and market penetration. An innovation in both access and pricing, this mechanism secured growth to over 100,000 treatments in 1 year.

Thomas pointed out that South Africa demonstrated what can be accomplished by using political will, a strong medical system willing to advance the standards of care, and broad engagement with private-sector implementing partners. Pharmaceutical companies cannot accomplish such work on their own; they need the help of other sectors. Thomas called for a needs-based approach to address issues in medical education; patient and consumer education; consumer-centered design; and simplification in the testing, diagnosis, and care pathway, as well as other health needs such as adequate nutrition that affects whether a medical intervention will have a successful outcome. Noting the years required to conduct TB trials, Thomas highlighted the need for the generation of reliable real-world evidence. Data on an intervention's effect on disease relapse after 100 weeks of treatment inherently calls for a long follow-up period. He suggested that the use of credible real-world cohorts could generate useful interim data. Successful regional efforts, such as those from South Africa, should be used globally. The Global Fund and J&J are currently conducting case-finding pilots in Indonesia and the Philippines. The company is forming similar partnerships in Russia and the Commonwealth of Independent States (CIS), and they are partnering with NGOs in China, India, and other parts of Southeast Asia. Building on what they learned from the MTV Staying Alive Foundation, J&J is carrying out a mass media campaign on social media and mainstream broadcast media in India to destigmatize TB and demonstrate the improvements in outcomes that are possible.

Implementing a New Treatment Regimen for Drug-Resistant Tuberculosis: Lessons Learned

Presented by Norbert Ndjeka, National Department of Health, South Africa

Ndjeka discussed the planning and implementation of a new shorter treatment regimen for DR TB—bedaquiline—in South Africa, with a focus on the factors that contributed to its success as well as the challenges that were encountered.

Drug-Resistant Tuberculosis in South Africa and the Effect of COVID-19

South Africa has one of the highest burdens of DR TB in the world, said Ndjeka. More than 13,000 cases of rifampicin-resistant (RR TB) and MDR TB were diagnosed in the country in 2019. During the same year, the estimated global incidence of RR TB and MDR TB was about 465,000 (WHO, 2020). Moreover, South Africa also has a high burden of HIV. Ndjeka noted that three-quarters of people with MDR TB in the country are also living with HIV, putting substantial pressure on systems of care for TB. However, despite South Africa's burden of DR TB, it outperforms the global rate for DR TB treatment initiation by almost twofold (WHO, 2020). In 2019, more than 9,000 people in the country were initiated on treatment for RR TB and MDR TB—including 406 cases of XDR TB[29]—representing 70 percent of all DR TB cases nationwide that year. Globally, about 177,000 patients began treatment for RR TB and MDR TB in 2019, representing around 38 percent of MDR TB cases.

Success rates for the treatment of DR TB in South Africa are also relatively high and have recently exceeded the global averages for both MDR TB and XDR TB (WHO, 2020). In 2017, the success rate for treatment of RR TB and MDR TB was approximately 60 percent in South Africa, surpassing the global rate of about 57 percent. The success rate for patients started on second-line treatment for XDR TB in 2016 in South Africa and worldwide were 60 percent and 47 percent, respectively.

Unfortunately, DR TB case-finding rates in South Africa have substantially declined since the onset of the COVID-19 pandemic, said Ndjeka. Between 2019 and 2020, the number of DR TB cases diagnosed dropped by 27 percent (2019: 11,274 cases; 2020: 8,229 cases), and this trend is predicted to continue through 2021. He posited that the nationwide lock-

---

[29] XDR TB is a type of MDR TB that is resistant to isoniazid and rifampicin, plus any fluoroquinolone and at least one of three injectable second-line drugs—amikacin, kanamycin, and/or capreomycin. See https://www.cdc.gov/tb/publications/factsheets/drtb/xdrtb.htm (accessed December 31, 2021).

downs implemented to control the pandemic have been a major contributing factor, but more research will be needed to fully understand the effect of the pandemic on the country's TB control program.

Planning and Implementing the Bedaquiline Clinical Access Programme in South Africa

Ndjeka provided an overview of the planning and implementation of the Bedaquiline Clinical Access Program in South Africa between 2011 and 2015, highlighting components that could potentially inform the rollout of novel shorter treatment regimens in other settings (Ndjeka et al., 2020). The first step was to establish a collaborative public–private working group that included representation from the national government, J&J, NGOs, and academia. This consortium led efforts to develop study protocols, obtain university ethics approval, engage with the medical product regulatory authority of South Africa (the Medicines Control Council), deliver training in both leadership and good clinical practice, engage with stakeholders across multiple sectors, and communicate with the managers of provincial TB programs. In addition to in-country work, the consortium also engaged with similar working groups around the world to better understand how to effectively roll out a new therapeutic and garner the necessary support. After developing the Bedaquiline Clinical Access Program, it was first implemented at five clinical sites prior to wider scale-up to additional sites.

Ndjeka remarked that numerous stakeholders and sectors are involved in implementing a new DR TB treatment regimen, such as the national and provincial TB programs, regulatory and ethics bodies, medicine procurement bodies, laboratory services, data management, and various national and international partners. Thus, a strong champion is needed to harmonize and lead the collaborative effort in addition to guidance from an expert committee. For example, because provinces in South Africa have a level of autonomy similar to U.S. states, gaining provincial-level buy-in for the bedaquiline rollout was also important.

Training of health care workers was central to the successful implementation of bedaquiline in South Africa, said Ndjeka. Treatment guidelines had to be revised to accommodate the new therapeutic regimens. Tools also needed to be aligned with those revisions and with the assessment of training needs. He noted that South Africa did not have sufficient resources to deliver trainings and obtain tools—for example, those used to detect adverse events, such as ECG and audiometers. However, various partnerships contributed funding and resources to provide training, acquire tools, and monitor training and results on the ground.

Robust cross-sector coordination across the government, academia, pharmaceutical sector, and finance sectors was another pillar of the rollout of bedaquiline, said Ndjeka. Strong political commitment from the national government—driven by strong engagement by the minister of health—was fundamental in gaining public buy-in and garnering resources to support the effort. The pharmaceutical sector provided support in procurement of medicines and other facets of supply chain management, while NGOs and academia provided technical support for the decentralized rollout of bedaquiline to provinces and districts.

Ndjeka emphasized that partnerships were critical in the implementation process. These partnerships facilitated the establishment of a broad network for diagnosing and treating MDR TB patients, as well as managing adverse events. For instance, the extent to which ototoxicity is an issue in managing MDR TB patients was initially underestimated, but this was better understood after most of the implementation sites were provided with portable audiometers. Partners also provided resources and support to improve electronic recording and reporting systems and to train health care workers on data and treatment management.

Factors Contributing to Success in Implementation

Ndjeka outlined several factors that contributed to the success in implementing the Bedaquiline Clinical Access Program. He extolled the benefits of a functional national committee bolstered by province-level clinical and programmatic subteams, as well as effective coordination between the National TB Program and the expert committee. Cooperation with the regulatory authority and other government sectors helped to streamline amendments to study protocols, for example. Initially the program was able to acquire the first round of doses through donation from J&J but later began purchasing doses directly. Developing a functional data system and effective laboratory services contributed to more accurate diagnostics, recording, reporting, and monitoring. The program also benefited from the availability of funds to convene various events to deliver trainings and share best practices. He highlighted a set of major lessons learned during the bedaquiline rollout that could be applicable to similar efforts in other settings (see Box 4-2).

Challenges Encountered in Implementation

Various challenges were encountered during the bedaquiline rollout in South Africa, said Ndjeka. At the early stages, it was challenging to secure buy-in from key stakeholders and manage their resistance to change. Obtaining regulatory authority for a new therapeutic is a lengthy process—even if only an amendment or new protocol is needed—that can delay implementation. Quantification and stock management pose additional challenges. For instance, scaling up bedaquiline in South Africa required running down and/

> **BOX 4-2**
> **Lessons Learned from the Rollout of Bedaquiline in South Africa**
>
> 1. Planning ahead is critical.
> 2. Foster interaction across government sectors responsible for acquiring drugs, laboratory supplies, and equipment.
> 3. Fulfill regulatory authority requirements.
> 4. Forge strong partnerships with academia, nongovernmental organizations, and the private sector.
> 5. Establish a national team to support clinical and programmatic activities.
> 6. Revise treatment guidelines.
> 7. Train health care workers.
> 8. Focus on innovation to adapt to unexpected changes.
>
> SOURCE: Presented by Norbert Ndjeka on September 15, 2021.

or writing off the large existing stock of existing drugs such as kanamycin. Moreover, it is challenging to ensure that the new regimen is being used universally in the field and to trace patients who may have been unnecessarily initiated on older injectable regimens. He also noted that the COVID-19 lockdown reduced the numbers of patients attending and presenting for care, and it may be difficult to re-engage them in treatment.

Effect of Bedaquiline Implementation

Ndjeka presented data on the DR TB treatment initiation, outcomes, and success rates in South Africa before and after the implementation of bedaquiline.[30] Between March 2013 and March 2015, 1 percent of all DR TB patients on treatment received the bedaquiline regimen (200/24,688 patients). Between March 2015 and December 2015, that proportion had risen to 12 percent (1,239/10,001) and by 2016, it had grown to 25 percent (2,973/11,994 patients). In 2017, the proportion of DR TB patients on treatment who were receiving the bedaquiline regimen reached 77 percent (8,240/10,754 patients).

DR TB treatment outcomes in South Africa improved markedly between 2010 and 2018 after the introduction of bedaquiline, particu-

---

[30] Bedaquiline received approval from the U.S. Food and Drug Administration in December 2012: https://www.jnj.com/media-center/press-releases/fda-grants-accelerated-approval-for-sirturo-bedaquiline-as-part-of-combination-therapy-to-treat-adults-with-pulmonary-multi-drug-resistant-tuberculosis (accessed December 31, 2021).

larly for patients with XDR TB. During that period, the treatment success rate for patients with XDR TB increased from 10 percent to 61 percent, while the death rate decreased from 49 percent to 21 percent. For MDR TB patients, the treatment success rate rose from 51 percent to 65 percent and the death rate declined slightly, from 19 percent to 17 percent. Among all patients initiated on treatment for DR TB in South Africa in 2017, a bedaquiline-containing regimen had a treatment success rate of 70 percent and death rate of 13 percent. In contrast, a non–bedaquiline-containing regimen (i.e., an older regimen consisting of injectable drugs) in the same cohort had a treatment success rate of 53 percent and a death rate of 23 percent. Ndjeka described these results as encouraging and catalytic for continued improvement.[31]

Bringing Innovation to the Development of New Transformative Tuberculosis Regimens

Presented by David Hermann, Bill & Melinda Gates Foundation

Hermann highlighted progress toward a shorter, simpler, safer pan-TB regimen—that is, a regimen for treating multiple forms of TB. He highlighted the R&D activities for TB over the past decade that are spurring progress toward a shorter, simpler, safer pan-TB regimen, which included the first approvals for several new TB drugs—bedaquiline, delamanid, and pretomanid—in a number of years. In 2020, the TBTC Study 31/A5349 and TB Alliance's Nix-TB bedaquiline-pretomanid-linezolid trial indicated that shortened TB course treatments are feasible. He emphasized the importance of this milestone, noting that years ago, regimen shortening was considered impossible because of the slow-growing nature of the TB bacteria. Moreover, adequate substrate for the R&D pipeline has been established and the new candidates bedaquiline, delamanid, pretomanid, sutezolid, and a decaprenylphosphoryl-ß-D-ribose-2'-oxidase (DprE1) inhibitor being developed by Otsuka Pharmaceutical may lead to the first generation of pan-TB regimens. At the same time, the COVID-19 pandemic has caused R&D disruptions such as closure of laboratories and clinics, which paused discovery research programs and clinical trial enrollment. While much TB research had resumed by the time of this workshop, the previous momentum has not yet been fully regained, said Hermann.

---

[31] Bedaquiline, though successful, has experienced slow rollout in sub-Saharan Africa owing to limited funding.

Optimal Pan-Tuberculosis Target Regimen Profile

Achieving a considerable decrease in TB incidence will involve transformative regimens that offer substantive improvements and help minimize the efficacy–effectiveness gap.[32] Although the results in clinical trials using the standard of care are promising, numerous factors create an efficacy–effectiveness gap, including tolerability, long duration of regimens, and the need for drug-susceptibility testing. Hermann explained that the target regimen profile (TRP) features a pan-TB product that does not require drug-susceptibility testing, has a shortened duration of 2 months or less, and is well-tolerated and affordable (see Table 4-1). Coupling this TRP with an improved point-of-care diagnostic would enable a pivot toward a "test and treat" paradigm in which a patient could be rapidly diagnosed and provided with pills in the same visit, leading to a high cure rate. He acknowledged the difficulty in fully achieving this scenario, and suggested that regimens that fall short of this aspirational goal could still be highly effective in the field. For example, the Nix-TB bedaquiline-pretomanid-linezolid regimen showed an efficacy rate of over 90 percent in the hardest-to-treat patients.

The goal of meeting the pan-TB TRP faces a number of challenges, Hermann noted. Although the portfolio of TB drugs is more vibrant and diverse in size and scope than ever before, antimicrobial candidates remain too few in number to achieve the TRP. More work is needed in discovery to identify novel drug targets to create more effective treatment combinations. Additionally, translational science is limited, and innovation is needed in biomarkers, dose selection, and efficient experimental design. Furthermore, quantitative translational modeling could be used. Continuing to establish connections between nonclinical tools, pharmacometrics modeling, and success in the clinic, as described by Nahid earlier from the experience with TBTC Study 31/A5349, would be beneficial. The TB toolbox is fairly extensive, and as more evaluations of regimens in the clinic are conducted, the tools that are essential in driving decision making can be identified. Hermann stated that no single organization will own the best candidates to build the most effective regimen, and therefore collaboration in TB R&D is critical. In working toward an aspirational TRP, the perfect should not be made the enemy of the good, he said. The focus should not be on finding a perfect nonclinical package that might translate into a regimen that meets TRP. Instead, good regimens with the potential to meet TRP should be moved into clinics in order to collect clinical outcomes data and translate this back to nonclinical results, said Hermann.

---

[32] The efficacy–effectiveness gap refers to the difference in observed outcomes in a controlled trial and those observed in clinical practice.

TABLE 4-1 Optimal Pan-Tuberculosis Target Regimen Profile

Target Regimen Profile Criteria	Hypotheses
Pan-tuberculosis	No drug-susceptibility testing required Fewer patients lost to the system after diagnosis
Shorter (<2–3 months)	Shorter → Improves adherence → Improves outcome → Less transmission
Safe and well-tolerated	No baseline or ongoing safety monitoring Well-tolerated → Improves adherence
Simpler	All oral; once-daily dosing, no drug–drug interactions to manage
Efficacious	Short, forgiving regimen noninferior to standard of care to minimize the efficacy–effectiveness gap
Affordable	Low barrier to uptake

SOURCE: David Hermann workshop presentation, September 15, 2021.

Innovation in Mycobacterium Tuberculosis *Antimicrobial Discovery*

Innovation is currently taking place in the area of *Mycobacterium tuberculosis* antimicrobial discovery, Hermann noted. For instance, clustered, regularly interspaced short palindromic repeats—known as CRISPR—interference was used as a platform to aid in lead target generation (Bosch et al., 2021). This platform was designed to allow titration of gene expression from full strength to virtually eliminated in a high-throughput in vitro system. This graded gene expression allows for measurement of bacterial fitness in vitro. Graphing the relationship between the magnitude of gene inhibition and cell fitness demonstrates that for some genes, a slight lowering in expression can have a profound effect on bacterial fitness, while others can be virtually knocked out with very little effect on fitness of the bacteria. The data derived from this system are used to create a vulnerability index for the potential target genes. Currently, the vulnerability index is being used by the TB Drug Accelerator (TBDA), a collaboration that focuses on drug discovery, to prioritize targets for TB discovery efforts. For example, transfer RNA synthetases and the DNA polymerase dnaE1 have distinguished themselves from other targets and are therefore receiving additional research focus, Hermann shared.

Innovation in Dose Selection

Hermann remarked that effective dosing is essential for any antibiotic, and particularly for a combination of drugs to treat TB. This disease results in complex, heterogeneous pathology; therefore, estimating the human dose across different sites of infection is challenging. Current research is generating pharmacokinetic and pharmacodynamic data across different sites of infection—plasma, lung, cell lesion, caseous lesion, cavity wall, and lymph node—in a rabbit model (Lakshminarayana et al., 2015). These data are used to estimate the human dose needed to provide lesion coverage, which is more difficult for drug penetration than other sites of infection. Hermann explained that if researchers focused on the plasma concentration to calculate the total dosing, appropriate lesion coverage would only be provided for a fraction of the overall dosing interval. Therefore, data on various infection sites are being used in the development of new TB drugs.

Collaboration is a key component in the R&D landscape. The European Regimen Accelerator for Tuberculosis program from the Innovative Medicines Initiative (IMI) is focused on early, preclinical, and phase 1 drug development, said Hermann. A company can set forth a new molecule, and the IMI will help drive it through the characterization of the early asset. Further downstream, IMI's UNITE4TB will then carry the work through phase 2. He noted that the Bill & Melinda Gates Foundation also sponsors similar collaborations through the TBDA, which has been active for 10 years and is a lead identification and optimization platform (Aldridge et al., 2021). Also downstream, the PAN-TB collaboration is composed of the TB Alliance, GlaxoSmithKline, J&J, Evotech, Otsuka, and the Gates Medical Research Institute. Hermann remarked that these collaborations drive the portfolio forward, and that data sharing is fundamental to this effort. Therefore, the Bill & Melinda Gates Foundation has embedded a basic tenet of data sharing in their investments that applies across organizations within a collaboration and across collaborations. Thus, the IMI collaborations work closely with PAN-TB and TBDA. Furthermore, the Critical Path Institute is a mechanism for sharing data with external partners.

Collaborating to Drive Innovation

Hermann highlighted innovation born of these collaborations, including work from PAN-TB on designing phase 2 trials to de-risk phase 3 trials. Hermann explained that drug developers may be wary of entering a 500-patient study with little additional clinical data. In one of the efforts to address this, PAN-TB is examining a stage design for a phase 2 trial through a pilot evaluation that studies the safety, tolerability, and trajectory of response for various TB regimens. This is a duration-finding study where a new regimen is dosed at different durations and the relationship between the regimen duration and outcomes is examined.[33] The study compares the trajectory

---

[33] Hermann noted that this innovative design builds off the work of many others, including Michael Hoelscher, German Center for Infection Research; the European and Developing Countries Clinical Trials Partnership; and Patrick Phillips and Rada Savic, Center for Tuberculosis at the University of California, San Francisco, among others.

of response for the standard of care with the trajectory for new regimens. Should a new regimen shorten the time in which the response trajectory moves from unfavorable to favorable status, these data can be used to de-risk the next stage of investment.

While much growth and progress have occurred in TB R&D, it has been slowed by the COVID-19 pandemic, said Hermann. However, the TB community is encouraged by current innovation and the potential PAN-TB studies that are staged to launch. The substrate for potentially effective regimens has been established and will continue to grow. Hermann remarked that this research warrants global engagement and funding comparable to that given to COVID-19.

Economic Analysis of Novel Tuberculosis Treatment Regimens

Presented by Anna Vassall, London School of Hygiene & Tropical Medicine

Vassall explored the value of conducting context-specific economic analyses of novel TB treatment regimens to inform future program design and investment. She explained that in the TB field, the conventional approach adopted by researchers is to perform economic analyses after positive trial results—such as those from TBTC Study 31/A5349, described by Nahid—with the aims of disseminating the results and convincing policy makers that the regimen is not only clinically effective, but also cost-effective, to promote funding and uptake. She offered an alternative perspective from a stakeholder who will fund the scale-up of a novel TB treatment regimen—particularly in low- and middle-income countries. Typically, the payer's goals are to use funding to (1) improve health-sector equity and efficiency, (2) strengthen the systems that are being implemented to inform priority setting within health sectors, and (3) conduct sectoral- and population-level economic analyses, which may be slightly different than economic analysis of an individual trial. Given the consistent lack of funding for TB over the past 20 to 30 years, understanding how that sectoral process works is pivotal to designing economic analyses that are more aligned with goals of payers, examining why uptake of a new regimen may be limited and potentially informing intervention design. Vassal explored how these systems for setting national priorities are evolving, with a focus on national-level payers and development partners—and reflected upon why previously effective TB interventions have not been funded to scale. She also discussed the specific case of shortened and universal TB regimens and aspects of the analyses that may be particularly promising.

Evolution of National Priority-Setting Systems Toward National Benefits Packages

Vassall provided an overview of the evolution of the systems for setting national priorities over the past decade, during which time many countries have created national strategic health plans that typically span from 3 to 5 years. Traditionally, people working in TB have focused on two strategies: garnering funding for new TB regimens within those national strategic plans sufficient for scaling up to high levels of coverage, and obtaining development assistance through various types of funding applications. However, the focus has shifted over the past 5 years toward universal health care (UHC) benefit packages, which involves examining the services that health sectors provide and defining the packages of care that should be publicly funded. This movement toward UHC benefit packages frames efforts to strengthen the health sector less in terms of how to plan finances for scale-up within 3 to 5 years and more in terms of whether a given intervention should be publicly funded at all. A component of this approach is to use a formal process of health technology assessment to evaluate new interventions or technologies in a way that extends beyond traditional guideline-type evaluation processes to consider cost-effectiveness within a local context. Vassall noted that several countries with high TB burdens have been embarking on this process of developing UHC benefits packages (e.g., Pakistan, India, Ethiopia) and others have already initiated health technology assessments around the rollout of national health insurance (e.g., China, India, South Africa, Ethiopia, Ghana, Kenya).

Inclusion of Tuberculosis Treatment in National Benefits Packages

As an example of how new TB treatment regimens can fit within national benefits packages, Vassall described cost-effectiveness analyses conducted in Ethiopia and Pakistan to inform which interventions would be included in their essential health packages. In Ethiopia, 159 health interventions were analyzed to determine which would be included as public-sector provisions (Eregata et al., 2021). Although various TB interventions analyzed were found to be less cost-effective than reproductive maternal and child health interventions and interventions for other infectious diseases, such as antiretroviral therapy for HIV, Ethiopia nonetheless decided to include most of the TB interventions in their intentionally ambitious package. However, the resulting package is unaffordable in many respects, necessitating priority setting that may delay the immediate inclusion of those TB interventions in practice.

Pakistan has adopted a more conservative approach to the inclusion of TB interventions in its benefits package by attempting to plan within its relatively limited fiscal space—the amount of financing that is actually available for the government to spend in the coming years—of just $8 dollars per capita at the district level to deliver an entire range of health services.[34,35] According to Vassall, a cost-effectiveness analysis of the district-level Essential Package Health Services in Pakistan found that the current treatment for DS TB is ranked 11th at $17 per disability-adjusted life year (DALY) averted. Even if that regimen becomes slightly more expensive, it is still affordable within the current fiscal space. In contrast, the current treatment for DR TB—which costs $757 per DALY averted—could only be afforded if there were increased expenditure. Vassall noted that from a human rights perspective, TB treatment should be considered in the context of other interventions. For example, the COVID-19 vaccine, at $6 per DALY averted, ranks 72nd in terms of cost-effectiveness and is considered affordable within Pakistan's current fiscal space. In a limited fiscal space, there is a trade-off between including a greater number of TB interventions in benefits packages regardless of their cost-effectiveness—and consequently achieving low coverage of all of them—versus including a smaller number of only the most cost-effective interventions and achieving full coverage.

Economic Assessment of Shortened Tuberculosis Treatment Regimens

Most analyses examining noninferior DS TB and DR TB regimens have found shortened regimens to be either cost saving or highly cost-effective at prices of around $1 to $5 per day compared to standard of care, said Vassall.[36] A caveat is that these analyses typically presume that DR TB treatment is fully financed, yet it is unclear whether even shorter regimens for DR TB would fit within the available fiscal space in many countries. Moreover, most of these modeling studies are based on limited direct effect on outcomes and trends transmission (i.e., 1–4 percent incidence). However, these savings could create considerably more potential for indirect health improvement for TB patients than if that funding were spent elsewhere. A moderately priced 4-week DS TB regimen would yield a 60 percent reduction in costs, both to health services and to patients. In absolute terms, the gains mainly accrue for households of patients with DS TB, because the cost per patient is much greater than the cost incurred by health services for each case of DS TB.

Such cost-efficiency gains to health systems are highly dependent upon context-specific factors, such as guideline adherence, the cost of current

---

[34] Vassall noted that prior to the COVID-19 pandemic, it was estimated that this amount would grow maximally to $12 dollars per capita, but given the fiscal situation in Pakistan and the effects of the pandemic, there is unlikely to be much growth from $8 dollars per capita.
[35] Costs in this analysis are given in U.S. dollars.
[36] Costs in this analysis are given in U.S. dollars.

delivery, and the baseline level of default. She noted that new regimens tend to yield fewer benefits when they are implemented within TB care systems that are already efficient compared with when implemented within less efficient systems. Additionally, the baseline level of treatment default can also underlie large differences in both outcome and costs. For example, the current delivery in Bangladesh was already cost-efficient and community based, so the cost savings for the community appear dampened compared with other settings. The experience in South Africa also demonstrates that guideline adherence—or the extent to which treatment is observed by health care workers—will determine the amount of treatment cost savings.

Pricing for a Future Universal Drug Regimen

Vassall and colleagues have looked ahead to 2030 to examine the pricing and value of a shortened universal drug regimen for TB when it eventually comes to market.[37] They considered the effect of changes in the size of the future fiscal space, the uptake of health technology assessments, and implementation of national strategic plans in the current planning and TB programs to estimate the potential revenues that would occur when those drugs were introduced. The price of the drug was estimated as the maximum price that would still ensure that the new TB regimen would fall into the package at that time, given the fiscal space available; that price was used to estimate revenues.

The modeling for India found that—depending upon the introduction of vaccines—higher revenues would be generated around treatment if the program performs well and creates more access to TB services, as intended over the next 10 years. Researchers also looked at the gain or loss in terms of price if the program does not achieve that level of performance—meaning, how the maximum price that could be charged would be affected by different regimen characteristics—and estimated the following maximum regimen prices (in U.S. dollars):

- Universal drug regimen, no drug-susceptibility testing requirement, 2-month duration, but laboratory monitoring required: $485.86.
- Two-month duration, no laboratory monitoring, but not universal (XDR not eligible), and drug-susceptibility testing required: $376.79.
- Universal drug regimen, no drug-susceptibility testing requirement, no laboratory monitoring, but 6-month duration: $112.47.

---

[37] This is ongoing, unpublished work from Vassall and colleagues.

Effect of Tuberculosis on Household Economic Status

The greatest economic gains from improvements in TB treatment and care are likely to be experienced by patients and their households in terms of protection from catastrophic expenditure and poverty, said Vassall. The effect of TB on the economic status of households is now well established. For instance, a modeling study estimated how many cases of poverty would be averted in India and South Africa by improvements in different types of TB treatments, finding a substantial increase in the number of households that would be pulled out of poverty (Verguet et al., 2017). However, she acknowledged that such arguments from the economic perspective do not necessarily appeal to the health-sector payer. In fact, there is an ongoing debate within health economics over whether health sectors should consider this type of information when allocating funding. To address this issue, Vassall and colleagues are exploring how to use economic evidence to make the case for investing in TB to ministries of finance and other non-health ministries who may be more interested in achieving poverty-reduction goals than specific TB-related health goals. The approach will vary by setting, but researchers are looking at how to integrate different types of modeling (e.g., return on investment, computable general equilibrium economic modeling) to effectively engage with stakeholders within ministries of finance.

Strategies for Using Economic Analyses of New Tuberculosis Regimens

Vassall highlighted several strategies for using economic analyses of new TB regimens to inform program design and garner investment in TB treatments and care. Cost-effectiveness analyses have long been used informally in this area, but formal cost-effective evidence is increasingly required. This work would benefit from a more comprehensive understanding of where TB currently sits, in terms of comparative efficiency, within the health sectors and how that varies by context and setting. Specifically, it is important to understand the cost gains that could be achieved with shortened TB regimens and in which countries those regimens would have the greatest effect. She noted that for DR TB treatments, those cost gains may enable scale-up, although that is likely to be different for DS TB treatments. A clear economic case can be made in terms of poverty reduction, but more work remains to elucidate how to make strong arguments to transform that evidence into investment by policy makers. She also underscored the value of using evidence brokers to inform investments and of empowering stakeholders working on the clinical and programmatic sides to optimize the use of economic evidence.

provide a systematic way to use the available data to track a country's progress toward major global TB targets, such as USAID strategy targets and UN high-level targets (see Figure 4-4). To help contextualize a country's status on key TB indicators, the PBMEF provides (1) a set of standardized indicators to measure essential TB program outputs and outcomes; (2) details on the performance of TB programs in specific technical areas (e.g., diagnosis, treatment, TB/HIV, private sector), and (3) treatment cascades and patient pathways for identifying gaps and needed improvements. A benefit is that using the framework does not require any substantial investment in collecting additional data; the available data are simply repackaged and used to monitor programs and inform decision making.

Core Indicators

The framework includes 10 core indicators (see Box 4-3) that capture fundamental elements of USAID's TB strategy—Reach, Cure, Prevent, and Sustain—and more than 180 extended indicators that fall under 14 technical

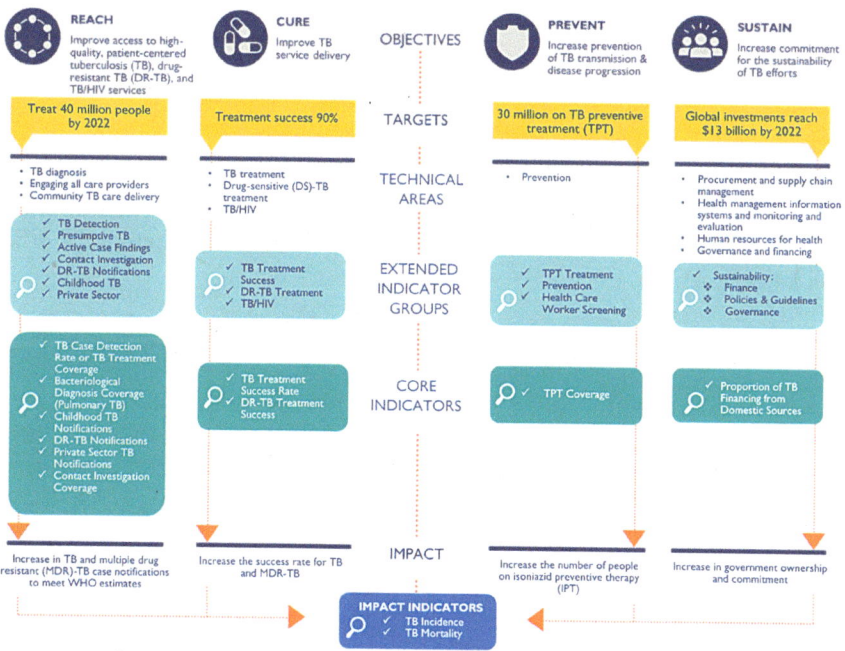

FIGURE 4-4 USAID's Performance-Based Monitoring and Evaluation Framework.
NOTE: WHO = World Health Organization.
SOURCE: Presented by Ezra Shimeles Tessera on September 15, 2021.

> **BOX 4-3**
> **Performance-Based Monitoring and Evaluation Framework: Core Indicators**
>
> 1. Tuberculosis (TB) case detection rate or TB treatment coverage
> 2. Bacteriological diagnosis coverage (pulmonary TB)
> 3. Childhood TB notifications
> 4. Drug-resistant TB notifications
> 5. Private-sector TB notifications
> 6. Contact investigation coverage
> 7. TB treatment success rate
> 8. Drug-resistant TB treatment success
> 9. TB preventive treatment coverage
> 10. Percentage of TB financing expected from domestic sources
>
> SOURCE: Presented by Ezra Shimeles Tessera on September 15, 2021.

categories. For instance, under the Reach domain are indicators that pertain to TB case-finding activities; under Cure are indicators related to treatment success; under Prevent are indicators tracking progress in infection control and delivering TB preventive therapy; and under Sustain are indicators covering financing, policies, guidelines, and governance. The PBMEF is a living document that can be continuously updated, harmonized, and adapted to individual country contexts and needs, he added. The core indicators are collected and used for monitoring, informing programmatic decision making, and facilitating collaboration with academics, researchers, and other technical partners.

Disease Cascade Analyses

The data collected using PBMEF indicators are also used to construct cascade analyses, said Tessera. For instance, USAID researchers have developed an HIV/TB infection cascade designed to help identify missing cases and—more importantly—to understand why they were missed in order to improve the system. If the core indicators are not sufficient to provide that insight, then extended indicators can contribute to a more in-depth and holistic analysis of the situation. Similarly, USAID has developed a cascade for DS TB disease that begins with an assessment of TB incidence in a population and then flows down through the numbers of individuals who (1) are eligible for screening, (2) have been screened, (3) have been evaluated, (4) have accessed a WHO-recommended rapid diagnostic test, (5) have bacteriologically confirmed pulmonary TB, (6) have accessed a drug-susceptibility test, (7) have notified DS TB, (8) have started TB treatment, and (9) have been successfully treated.

Framing Tuberculosis as a Global Health Emergency
Presented by Richard Chaisson, Johns Hopkins University School of Medicine

Chaisson's presentation focused on the need to frame TB as a global health emergency. He noted that WHO declared TB a global public health emergency in 1993 (Nakajima, 1993) and declared COVID-19 a public health emergency of international concern on January 30, 2020.[39] Those declarations are the sole similarity between the global responses to these global health emergencies. The COVID-19 response from the scientific, public health, medical, and pharmaceutical communities has been spectacular in developing diagnostics, therapeutics, and vaccines at a dizzying pace, he remarked. The resulting armamentarium of tools provides the means to control and end the COVID-19 pandemic. Although the effective and equitable deployment of these tools remains a monumental challenge, science clearly answered the call of this global crisis. In contrast, TB has never been treated as a true global health emergency. This may be attributable to TB's long-standing history, the absence of a rapid escalation in case numbers, and the golden age of discovery in the twentieth century that has come and gone. However, the worldwide distribution of TB is just as great as that of COVID-19. Chaisson stated that TB's effects on health and survival are similarly dire, and the need for a rapid, coordinated, and adequately resourced scientific response is equally evident.

Treating an epidemic as an emergency generates substantive differences in response, as demonstrated by the response to COVID-19, stated Chaisson. The development of diagnostic tests for COVID-19 proceeded at near miraculous speed. Most academic medical centers in the United States and Europe established their own in-house diagnostic polymerase chain reaction tests within weeks. Referencing his work on a COVID-19 treatment trial with Novartis and the AIDS Clinical Trials Group funded by NIH, he described how the U.S. Food and Drug Administration (FDA) review, institutional review board (IRB) approval, and clinical launch of a phase 3 randomized, double-blind, placebo-controlled clinical trial for hydroxychloroquine

---

[39] See Statement on the second meeting of the International Health Regulations (2005) Emergency Committee regarding the outbreak of novel coronavirus (2019-nCoV), https://www.who.int/news/item/30-01-2020-statement-on-the-second-meeting-of-the-international-health-regulations-(2005)-emergency-committee-regarding-the-outbreak-of-novel-coronavirus-(2019-ncov) (accessed January 1, 2022).

and azithromycin all took place within 6 weeks. COVID-19 vaccines went from sequence to phase 1 in less than 8 weeks, moved to phase 3 about 4 months later, and were approved by the FDA within 11 months. Institutions treated COVID-19 as a crisis and operated in crisis mode, said Chaisson. For example, the IRB at Johns Hopkins University met 5 days per week to review COVID-19 protocols. NIH issued supplemental awards within 2 weeks, and $500 million was invested in diagnostics in less than 2 months.

Chaisson described TB vaccines as far more challenging to develop than those for COVID-19. In the absence of adequate investment and an emergency response, the pace of implementation of TB trials is slow. For instance, Johns Hopkins University is currently conducting a suite of studies funded by Unitaid to promote broader implementation of TB preventive therapy with short-course regimens. Chaisson recalled priorities outlined earlier in the workshop by Matteo Zignol, head of the Prevention, Care, and Innovation Unit of the Global TB Programme at WHO, noting that regulatory processes are delaying (1) trials on interactions of rifapentine and antiretroviral drugs in pregnant women and children infected with HIV, (2) implementation in high-burden settings, and (3) the use of short-course regimens in populations that have not yet been studied, such as household contacts. Review by the WHO Ethics Committee takes an average of 10 to 12 months. National IRBs in Brazil and India take up to a year. Although the United States conducts review processes in less time, the overall timeline for conducting TB research remains long. Treatment for TB is lengthy and endpoints are slow to accrue, leading to time-intensive TB clinical trials. However, TB studies are prolonged unnecessarily by a lengthy administrative and regulatory review process, he stated.

The problem is greater than the mechanics of any individual agency or body, Chaisson noted. Part of the issue is a lack of urgency around TB; the response to COVID-19 illustrates that when a disease is treated as an emergency, processes move rapidly. An example of the slow processes delaying TB trials is the 6-month time frame for an IRB review of a protocol amendment to take place. In addition, the research infrastructure—from investigators to IRBs to regulatory agencies—is underfunded and undersupported, said Chaisson. Just as individual research is underfunded, so too is the machinery of clinical research. The WHO Ethics Committee requires a year to review protocols owing to inadequate staffing and a reliance on volunteer reviewers who have other full-time jobs to perform. The trials for COVID-19 therapeutics and vaccines demonstrated that it is possible to conduct game-changing trials in record time without cutting corners when the situation is treated as an emergency and enormous human and financial resources are allocated to the emergency.

A twofold approach can be used to address regulatory issues hampering TB innovation, Chaisson stated. First, more investment is needed in regulatory and research ethics and administrative aspects of clinical research and clinical trials to ensure that requirements do not stifle innovative research.

Second, regulatory review could be streamlined to eliminate unnecessary processes that add delay while doing little to protect study participants or communities. For example, local institutions have a legal responsibility to protect research participants as they carry out IRB reviews, yet a WHO review is also conducted, adding little value to the process while causing substantial delays, said Chaisson. Advances in TB diagnosis, treatment, and prevention that will translate into progress in TB elimination could be pursued as an emergency. He stated that unless TB is treated as a global health emergency, advances in the development of tools to end TB will continue to be very slow, and unacceptably high rates of disease, suffering, and death will continue.

DISCUSSION

Strengthening the Tuberculosis Response

Gail Cassell, senior lecturer on global health and social medicine at Harvard Medical School, remarked that in her experience with TB, she has observed a lack of harmonization in regulatory processes, drug facilities and timing, and drug expiration, all of which create challenges. She suggested that the National Academy of Medicine consider a future workshop focused on the issue of regulatory harmonization with specific emphasis on TB. Kester commented that the science and technology needed to address many public health issues are relatively straightforward, and generating political will and investment is the major hurdle. However, TB also entails substantial development costs. Clinical trials for regulatory approval are expensive, and the cost of deployment is a challenge in its own right. Kester contrasted the attention given to TB—which has existed for a long time and is a huge global problem—with COVID-19, which is constantly featured in the news, and case counts by county are reported daily. He asked how the public can be sensitized to the huge public health issue that TB is in order to increase the rate of progress, which is currently very slow.

Chaisson replied that TB remains a long-standing, difficult problem to solve because of a general lack of concern about the disease. In 2020, COVID-19 surpassed TB as a global cause of death. Despite TB having killed more people than any other infection in history, it does not garner the attention that COVID-19 does. He stated that the governmental response to COVID-19 has been appropriate, but a similar response to TB is necessary. People do not view TB as an emergency right now, but this was the case even when it was declared an emergency 28 years ago. The current response to COVID-19 is unsustainable, said Chaisson. For instance, institutional review boards have become fully dedicated to COVID-19 trials while processes for other diseases are halted. He remarked that the approach taken with HIV is an example of a sustainable path forward. Grants related to HIV are prioritized, with the NIH review process for HIV taking 2 to 2.5 months, in comparison with 10 to 12 months for grants for TB and other conditions.

Chaisson explained that an HIV grant submitted in early September is typically reviewed by October or November and funded by January. Thus, implementation of interventions for HIV takes place more quickly than for other conditions. When an innovation such as dolutegravir—an antiretroviral medication used to treat HIV—becomes available, countries demand it, WHO recommends it, Unitaid funds expansion of its production, and it is implemented, he remarked. In contrast, implementation of innovations for TB such as bedaquiline—a drug used to treat MDR TB—can take many years. Chaisson said that people must care about TB in order to adequately address it, and the magnitude of the problem should be emphasized to make it more compelling. Wells remarked that creating a focus on TB and generating resources to address it is an ongoing challenge. Prior efforts include marketing XDR TB as "Ebola with wings" and connecting TB with HIV in the President's Emergency Plan for AIDS Relief.

Monique Mansoura, executive director for Global Health and Biotechnology at the MITRE Corporation, commented that coronavirus vaccine development was de-prioritized for 17 years. The 2003 emergence of severe acute respiratory syndrome (SARS) and its reemergence in 2012 were not met with aggressive action to address coronaviruses as a public health or national security threat. When taking a longer view of investment in coronaviruses, one can see passivity. She emphasized that the opportunities for collaboration and cost savings in addressing both TB and COVID-19 need to be recognized. Tackling TB builds the capabilities that have value in addressing future outbreaks, epidemics, and pandemics. Instead of positioning TB against other threats, the shared benefits of addressing all threats can be highlighted.

Data Sharing and Standardization

Kester asked how data sharing and standardization can be organized to generate data that can be compared across trials and across regions, and thus making it relevant for various future actions. Hermann replied that much progress is needed in TB's development as an R&D discipline. Inefficiencies occur when extracting information from across trials and also from translating nonclinical experimental models to clinical models. Data sharing is the only way to advance R&D progress, said Hermann. Both nonclinical and clinical trial data should be shared, and this presents challenges and legal aspects to consider. He noted that the Bill & Melinda Gates Foundation has a fundamental tenet of data sharing being the expectation, and all investments made by the foundation include data-sharing commitments. This has resulted in two TB investments in which patient-level data were aggregated through a data repository, and analysis of these pooled data led to insights. Hermann noted that data sharing is not easy, but it is possible, and important lessons can be derived from pooled analysis efforts.

Nahid remarked that some people question the value of data sharing in relation to the amount of effort it requires. He shared a recent experience in pooling the data from four fluoroquinolone-substitution trials. Even though these trials found the experimental 4-month regimens to be inferior, he and his colleagues were able to learn about disease phenotypes, the critical importance of standardizing TB outcomes, and the effect of nonadherence (Imperial et al., 2018). For example, they found that one of the biggest drivers of an unfavorable outcome was missing as few as 1 in 10 doses. This illustrates the value of pooling data for clinical applications, and this value extends to the preclinical space. Pooled data analysis de-risks decision making for the entire TB therapeutics community, said Nahid (Lienhardt and Nahid, 2019).

Considerations for Tuberculosis Research and Authorization

Cassell commented on how little was initially known about COVID-19, particularly in respect to its broad clinical manifestations and the long-term damage it can cause. Despite the virus not being fully understood, rapid developments took place to address COVID-19. Emergency authorizations were used to allow earlier approval of vaccines and treatments to combat COVID-19 while continuing to collect and analyze real-world data. If resources and time were unlimited, knowing everything possible about the pathogen before proceeding would be preferable. However, Cassell wondered if perhaps a lesson from this is that moving forward faster—without having all scientific questions answered first—may be beneficial in addressing infectious diseases, including TB, and whether the approach should be considered.

Chaisson remarked that clinical product development needs a foundation of robust basic research and discovery. He pointed to a 1992 commentary that identified TB as an emerging problem and described how TB research funding dwindled in the 1960s because of decades of disease decline in the United States (Bloom and Murray, 1992). He further noted that during his years at medical school, TB was only mentioned once during a pathology course and was omitted from all other courses, including microbiology. TB was no longer considered modern science at that time, he said. In the 1980s, Chaisson's chief of medicine tried to dissuade him from conducting research on TB in San Francisco residents with HIV. The research ethos around TB was deconstructed in the 1960s and has not been reconstructed since. Nonetheless, TB researchers today are taking up and using modern techniques. He noted that the Johns Hopkins University Center for Tuberculosis Research shares a building with cancer research labs, and he and his colleagues have found that TB research has much in common with cancer research and microbiome research, as they use similar methodologies. Product studies can identify new targets that inform the development of new medicines that eventually become the focus of clinical trials, he emphasized. Comprehensive basic science and pathogenesis research is being rebuilt, and this is necessary in advancing TB research, said Chaisson.

Translational Medicine and Human-Centered Design

Wells noted that workshop sessions have highlighted the role of translational medicine in TB innovation and discovery, in translation from the clinical trial to implementation, and in economics. A shorter regimen would be transformative for TB treatment, and efficient TB treatment could reduce poverty. He asked how much communication is needed between the upstream clinical space and the downstream implementation space as trials are designed and executed. Nahid replied that human-centered design, patient preference aspects, and program preference aspects are essential to incorporate in the early development of a new regimen or tool. He added that this is a growth area for the TB community. The WHO Guideline Development Committee approach to endorsing a regimen includes a multidimensional examination of benefits and harms that includes the patient experience of the implementation of the new regimen (WHO, 2014). Collecting data early in the design process can help WHO endorse and facilitate the scale-up of new designs.

Capacity for mRNA Technology and Vaccine Production

Schmidt remarked that more research on pathogenicity and antigen discovery is needed. He noted that with mRNA platforms, it is possible to express a dozen antigens easily, yet researchers do not know which antigens to express. Understanding the biology to guide development requires the investment of money and effort. Reed agreed that discovery of new target antigens is time-intensive, and delivery mechanisms can be developed in parallel. At the same time, the good should not be killed in search of the perfect, he emphasized, noting that a vaccine antigen that provides up to and beyond 50 percent protection can advance the goal of disease elimination. Cassell noted that Moderna announced that they will manufacture mRNA vaccines for HIV. She asked whether HDT Bio has a TB vaccine center in Rwanda. Reed replied that HDT Bio's most active center is in India, and the Indian and Korean centers have committed to providing vaccines to Africa. The organization seeded a pilot production facility in Cape Town several years ago, and this will be expanded to other countries—including Rwanda—to increase local capacity. The Korean facility is a modern factory built to manufacture recombinant TB vaccines. Although TB is not a major problem in Korea, the country is committed to addressing it and has invested heavily in the company. In fact, Korea has two state-of-the-art facilities: the recombinant vaccine technology center and a center for BCG vaccine funded in part by the Green Cross. Korea will assist HDT Bio in transferring technology once African sites have the ability to receive it, said Reed. He added that the focus in these sites should be on the infrastructure and training needed to receive and sustain local production capability. Brazil has all the components in place, including machines, good manufacturing practices, trained personnel, and funding. Reed stated the hope that Africa will likewise be able to establish capacity. He noted that discovery should continue, and it should focus on antigens as well as delivery mechanisms, as the delivery of an RNA or new antigen can increase the vaccine's efficacy.

Reflections on the Session

Kester remarked that the multipronged approaches presented at this workshop are promising, from the potential for new lessons in the use of well-characterized products such as BCG to the emerging RNA vaccine technology, given that they can be paired with political will and investment funding. COVID-19 has not only been the impetus for COVID-19 vaccines, it has accelerated new vaccine technology, including mRNA approaches. The COVID-19 pandemic has also sensitized policy makers and funders to the value of vaccines. He noted that not all vaccines will be able to be developed, tested, deployed, and approved in the shorter time frame in which COVID-19 vaccines were created. Researchers should guard against the perception that such a timeline is feasible for all vaccines. The continued demonstration of value of new adjuvants holds the potential to increase the efficacy of antigens via the appropriate adjuvant formulation. Kester commented that host-directed approaches and the interaction of pathogens with the host are areas meriting further study. The possibility of shortening the regimen holds promise, as data indicate that the long-held view that TB treatment must be slow and lengthy is not necessarily accurate. He noted that all approaches hold both risk and opportunity, and that the challenge is using the existing science rather than searching for the perfect solution.

Wells remarked that he has worked on TB for many years—seeing much transformation—and the current moment is unprecedented in terms of opportunity for innovation. At the same time, TB efforts have experienced setbacks because of COVID-19, particularly in terms of case finding. He stated that the rapid progress of development and innovation in finding new drugs and vaccines give him hope for TB. Although the disease is challenging to combat owing to its lower incidence in high-income countries, the TB research space is more active than ever before. Kenneth Castro, professor of global health, epidemiology, and infectious diseases at Emory University, added that the latest developments renew his optimism that advances can be achieved. The ball was dropped with TB, and now is the time to pick it up and use the current opportunities discussed at this workshop, he added.

Cassell noted that host-directed therapies, particularly Gleevec (imatinib), could offer a major advantage if they are able to act synergistically with antibiotics. This area warrants attention and could yield considerable advances, she believes. In addition, the IMPAc-TB study funded by the National Institute of Allergy and Infectious Diseases is examining immunological aspects of TB in a collaborative way that has not before been attempted. She emphasized that a vaccine that provides 50 percent protection can substantially curb the TB epidemic, and therefore technologies for these products should be advanced. Data indicates that via mRNA, a combination of antigens could help control TB and reduce the costs of doing so. Regulatory harmonization is an issue that should be addressed quickly to decrease the time it takes to receive WHO approval for manufacturing, said Cassell. She noted that in her experience, the approval process for companies to manufacture TB drugs can take up to 2 years; during that time, lives could be saved by the tried-and-true drugs awaiting approval.

5

Financing, Ambition, and Preparedness

The third session of the second part of the workshop explored strategies for eliminating tuberculosis (TB) in a global context dramatically changed by the COVID-19 pandemic. The session featured remarks by Tharman Shanmugaratnam, senior minister and coordinating minister for Social Policies of Singapore and co-chair of the G20 High-Level Independent Panel (HLIP) on Financing the Global Commons for Pandemic Preparedness and Response (PPR), in which he discussed the synergy involved in developing prevention and response efforts for TB and COVID-19 and summarized the HLIP's strategies for such efforts. A panel followed, moderated by Peter Sands, executive director of the Global Fund to Fight AIDS, Tuberculosis and Malaria (the Global Fund), that explored how efforts to combat TB can be incorporated into the global health security and pandemic preparedness agenda. Panelists included John Bell, Regius Professor of Medicine at Oxford University; Bruce Gellin, chief of Global Public Health Strategy for the Rockefeller Foundation's Pandemic Prevention Institute; Rebecca Katz, professor and director of the Center for Global Health Science and Security at Georgetown University; and Michael Callahan, clinical associate physician at Massachusetts General Hospital and president of the Division of Cellular Therapeutics at United Therapeutics. Margaret Hamburg, interim vice president of global biological policy and programs for the Nuclear Threat Initiative, moderated the second panel, which considered the economic rationale for financing the elimination of TB. The panelists were Mike Reid, assistant professor in the Department of Medicine at the University of California, San Francisco (UCSF), associate director of the UCSF Center for Global Health Delivery, Diplomacy, and Economics, and chief medical officer for the UCSF

Pandemic Initiative for Equity and Action; Bjørn Lomborg, president of the Copenhagen Consensus Center and visiting fellow at the Hoover Institution at Stanford University; Mark Dybul, chief executive officer of Enochian Biosciences, professor of medicine at Georgetown University, and former executive director of the Global Fund; and Amanda Glassman, executive vice president and senior fellow at the Center for Global Development and chief executive officer of the center's branch in Europe.

In his opening remarks, Sands described the Global Fund as the largest provider of external financing for TB interventions, contributing approximately 75 percent of the world's external TB financing. The organization's 2020 report outlines that for the first time in the 20-year history of the Global Fund's programmatic results, backslides occurred across all three diseases of HIV, TB, and malaria (Global Fund, 2021). The COVID-19 pandemic created massive disruptions in service provision and diverted human and financial resources, including laboratory capacity, from other diseases. Sands noted that of the three diseases of focus, TB efforts have been most undermined by COVID-19. From 2018 to 2020, the number of people treated for TB decreased by 1 million, representing an 18 percent decline in the number of cases being treated. Sands noted that this assuredly translates into hundreds of thousands of deaths. Thus, the COVID-19 pandemic has been a catastrophe on multiple fronts.

Disruption continued into 2021, said Sands. India's TB program was disrupted when the pandemic began in 2020, but began regaining momentum at the end of 2020 and the beginning of 2021, as evidenced by a sharp increase in TB case notification rates. However, the COVID-19 surge brought on by the Delta variant in the late spring and summer of 2021 once again disrupted TB interventions, despite efforts made by national television programs and civil society to mitigate the damage. Sands pointed out that pandemics affect TB, but TB can also affect preparedness against pandemics. The laboratory capacity, molecular testing instruments, and contact tracing systems developed for TB have been used to address COVID-19. Indeed, the established TB testing capacity served as the backbone of COVID-19 molecular testing activity in many countries. Furthermore, many leaders within the TB community have been called on to serve as leaders of national COVID-19 responses because of their expertise in respiratory diseases. Sands remarked that while TB may have the most to lose from COVID-19, it also has the most to contribute. The interconnection between fighting TB and making the world safer from future pathogen threats—particularly respiratory pathogens—should be explored.

Victor Dzau, president of the National Academy of Medicine, remarked on the devastating consequences of TB experienced by his grandparents, parents, and other relatives during his childhood in Asia. The Global Fund and the President's Emergency Plan for AIDS Relief (PEPFAR) have created resources for low-income countries so they can address chronic endemic and pandemic diseases. Although it was necessary to pivot these resources to COVID-19, this came at a cost in setting back TB elimination efforts, including testing and treatment. Dzau suggested that the pandemic preparedness effort should avoid investing in silos and instead invest in programs that strengthen countries' capacity to fight HIV, TB, and malaria. Building resilient health systems will provide better services for both TB and COVID-19 patients, he added.

A PLACE FOR TUBERCULOSIS IN THE PANDEMIC PREPAREDNESS AGENDA

Remarks by Tharman Shanmugaratnam, Co-chair, G20 High-Level Independent Panel

Tharman explored how to situate TB within the pandemic preparedness agenda. He noted that we are at an important juncture that has focused the world's attention on infectious disease threats. We have to fortify our own defenses in a way that addresses not just one disease or prospective new disease at a time but recognizes that we have a plethora of both existing diseases that are unchecked and potential new ones. The effort can no longer be easily compartmentalized into global regions either. For instance, evidence suggests that human incursions into the natural environment, the deterioration of biodiversity, and climate change are increasing the likelihood of zoonotic spillovers and a broader spread of vector-borne diseases. Infectious disease threats and climate change are the central challenges of our times for national and global governments, he added.

Intersection of Pandemic and Endemic Diseases

A major pandemic interacts with endemic diseases, resulting in cost to human life from the pandemic disease as well as from the significant diversion of resources away from the treatment of endemic diseases. In the case of the COVID-19 pandemic, TB has been the most prominent casualty, said Tharman. Around the world, a startling reduction in health care system access has occurred, with manpower and facility occupancy diverted toward COVID-19. The pandemic has also affected human behavior, with fear of contracting the disease increasing people's aversion to accessing medical treatment. Case notifications for TB significantly decreased throughout Asia in 2020 (WHO, 2021c), setting the stage for increases in TB cases and fatalities in the years to come. Thus, pandemic prevention and preparation is critical for limiting both the direct effects of the outbreak and the indirect effects resulting in neglect of treatment for other diseases. Additionally, the capacity to address endemic diseases—including surveillance systems for early detection, trained health workers in communities, and health care capabilities at the primary and tertiary levels—should be strengthened, recognizing the high degree of synergy between capabilities developed for endemic diseases and those required to treat a new pandemic.

Structural bias within the research and development (R&D) of treatments results in a commercial incentive to treat diseases prevalent in high-income countries versus diseases prevalent in low-income countries, observed Tharman. Once TB was no longer a major threat to high-income countries, the pharmaceutical industry and other groups that were engaged in R&D investment for vaccines and drugs had little commercial incentive to direct resources to TB. The bifurcated and inequitable nature of funding disease prevention and treatment is likely to decrease trust globally, he noted. The COVID-19 pandemic had seen a lack of access to lifesaving medical supplies in a large part of the developing world, putting this dynamic into sharp focus. He remarked that when combined with the continued inattention to endemic diseases, this lack of trust now risks becoming entrenched and more difficult to overcome. Thus, increased access to vaccines and other critical medical supplies required to address COVID-19 is an urgent need, as is acknowledging and treating endemic diseases in all regions of the world as important issues, said Tharman.

Elaborating on the lack of boundaries for infectious disease threats, he warned that the longer the pandemic spreads unchecked, the greater the risk that new COVID-19 variants will emerge. Likewise, the persistence of TB around the world coupled with improper use of drug treatments and inadequate testing is giving rise to drug-resistant TB, including multidrug-resistant TB (MDR TB). Continued neglect of TB control and improper treatment use could lead to an emergent pandemic of drug-resistant TB from which no part of the world is protected. Thus, he underscored the need for urgency in tackling COVID-19, preparing for future pandemics, and addressing endemic diseases—TB being foremost among them.

There is no lack of ambition in current plans, such as in the World Health Organization's (WHO's) End TB Strategy, which includes targets, pillars, and a multisectoral accountability framework (WHO, 2015). Tharman noted that other global health organizations—including the Global Fund, the Stop TB Partnership, and others—have also made meaningful advances in partnerships with one another and with employer groups and global funds. For instance, in 2020 the World Economic Forum, the Confederation of Indian Industry, Johnson & Johnson, Royal Philips, Fullerton Health, the Global Fund, and the Stop TB Partnership were involved in an initiative to address TB in the workplace.[1] However, a fundamental problem is lack of

---

[1] This initiative is called Ending Workplace TB. See https://www.ewtb.org (accessed January 1, 2022).

investment and financing for the TB eradication effort and for infectious disease threats more broadly, he added.²

Tharman remarked that we need a basic reset of the system to address the current gaps. This reset need not attempt a grand reconstruction of multilateralism, nor can it simply be about incremental changes in existing institutions, because the system is fragmented, dependent on bilateral contributions, reactive, and wholly inadequate. He envisions reforms to involve creative ways of strengthening multilateralism, improving existing bilateral initiatives, and simultaneously strengthening ways to address endemic threats and new health care security threats. The first step in this complex work is incentivizing national governments to increase activity in identifying and addressing infectious disease threats, said Tharman. This work has not been adequately prioritized in the budgets of a broad range of countries for a variety of reasons. Because infectious disease threats can cross borders, containing these threats is of national, regional, and global benefit, and is therefore a global public good. Therefore, financing systems should extend beyond domestic resource mobilization guidance to low-income countries; they should provide international support to incentivize investment in the capacities in these countries that carry international benefit. Tackling infectious disease threats should also not be limited to bilateral aid strategies. Instead, the issue should be framed as a matter of collective investment in global public goods that will benefit nations of all income levels, he added.

Strategy for Collective Investment in Global Public Goods

The G20 HLIP on Financing the Global Commons for PPR created a strategy for this collective investment that features key strategic moves (G20 HLIP, 2021). First, global health organizations require more reliable funding from both bilateral and multilateral sources in order to fulfill their missions, said Tharman. Stronger multilateral funding provided on a reliable basis is needed to address WHO's insecure financial footing. Global health organizations—including the Global Fund, the Global Alliance for Vaccines and Immunisation (Gavi), the Coalition for Epidemic Preparedness Innovations (CEPI), One Health Partners, and others—all require reliable funding to fully address their mandates.

The second strategy is to strengthen the role of international financial institutions (IFIs) in tackling infectious diseases. These institutions include the World Bank, the International Monetary Fund (IMF), various regional

---

² For more information on global targets for mitigating TB, see the following resources from the UN High-Level Meeting on the Fight Against TB (UNHLM TB): https://www.stoptb.org/advocacy-and-communications/unhlm-tb-key-targets-and-commitments.

development banks, and bilateral commercially oriented development banks that play useful roles in various regions. The IFIs have largely focused on country programs for country benefit. The context in which IFIs were founded led them to design programs at the national level addressing health care, education, infrastructure, and other areas. For instance, the World Bank and IMF were founded after World War II in response to issues surrounding economic reconstruction and balance of payments, which were countries' own internal problems. Tharman stated that the time has come to repurpose IFIs to address threats to the global commons, because tackling these threats—in addition to poverty eradication and ensuring inclusive growth—is the central challenge countries face. Addressing threats to the global commons requires investment in global public goods on a national and regional level and, to some extent, in global facilities and networks. This will require the World Bank and IMF to work with other multilateral development banks. Additionally, an increase in grant resources is needed to incentivize investment in capacity building. Commercial loans are inadequate, given that the rest of the world will derive benefit from these investments in low-income countries. Strengthening the role of IFIs in tackling infectious disease threats and, more generally, threats to the global commons will multiply capital for these endeavors, he remarked, by using resources of shareholders through the capital markets, as well as by incentivizing governments to do their part. Thus, repurposing IFIs for the current era is important in meeting the central challenge facing individual countries, that of threats to the global commons, he remarked.

The third strategic move is the creation of a new global financing mechanism that provides an overlay on the financing of individual organizations. The current system is gravely underfunded and unpredictably funded; it will not be repaired by increasing bilateral funding for existing institutions alone, said Tharman. A multilateral layer of financing is needed to work synergistically with the individual organizations that play critical roles in global health security. A challenge in creating such an overlay is avoiding further fragmentation or the introduction of new inefficiencies into the system. This can be accomplished with the creation of a global health threats fund. Rather than serve as an operational entity, this global health security fund would bring forth additional resources for existing organizations. For example, such a global health threats fund could provide additional resources to the International Development Association, the Global Fund, Gavi, or any other organization working to garner support for programs that deal with both emerging and existing threats, on the condition that the organization also used funds from bilateral or philanthropic sources. In other words, the multilateral fund would not divert resources that otherwise would have gone to existing organizations, but instead seek to supplement such funds.

Integrating Pandemic Preparedness and Endemic Disease Control

Efforts to prevent and prepare for future pandemics should be integrated with efforts to address endemic diseases to the fullest extent possible, Tharman stated. Preventing and preparing ourselves well for pandemics is critical not only in its own right but because of the much broader cost pandemics impose on society, not the least being the neglect of other pressing public health needs, he emphasized. The nature of the facilities and human resources required to address pandemics and endemics is the same. Efforts to contend with TB and other infectious diseases involve building the capability to detect, diagnose, and treat disease quickly. In addition, capacities such as global surveillance networks, data sharing, and genomic sequencing are in need of massive scaling up, he remarked.[3]

Currently, international, national, and regional facilities are underprepared. Resolving issues of supply capacity should aim to radically shorten the time required to roll out vaccines, therapeutics, personal protective equipment, and other critical supplies on a global scale. This increased capacity could be used in interpandemic years to meet the needs caused by endemic diseases and other public health requirements. Even excess capacity maintained for a future pandemic would be a worthwhile investment, as the funds spent on manufacturing capacity will be recouped many times over through the rapid delivery of critical supplies thus reducing the costs of a pandemic, he added. The most efficient preparation for future pandemics relies on and reinforces the work involved in tackling endemic diseases.

A new multilateral funding mechanism has the potential to strengthen multilateralism, achieve better synergy with bilateral efforts, and improve relationships between institutions to network more effectively and attack problems more seamlessly. The G20 HLIP estimated that a global health threats fund would require a minimum of $10 billion per year. Tharman remarked that although this figure sounds high, it is a small sum relative to the potential gains and to a country's ability to afford it. Spread out over countries, this figure comes to approximately 0.02 percent of gross domestic product (GDP), reflecting a small sum if distributed across countries on a fair and equitable basis. Thus, politics, not finance, is the constraint in moving this initiative forward.

Political will is needed to invest collectively in collective security. Investing in collective security is not only a global good, it is also for the good of each individual nation. Finance is not the constraint, but rather it is myopia in governance and politics that is causing the holdup in many parts of the

---

[3] The WHO supranational reference lab system works to expand and link TB genomic sequencing. See Gilpin and Mirzayev, 2019.

world; that is, the lack of recognition that one's own country's interests are best served through collective investment in collective health care security, and what is now needed is leadership to push this through. The $10 billion figure—a conservative estimate that does not take into account all the investments necessary—illustrates the gross underfunding of the system. Tharman noted that one of the few benefits of COVID-19 is that it has forced perspective shifts to an extent that past epidemics and pandemics did not. The current climate can be capitalized upon to make bold changes in international cooperation to preserve health security.

Discussion

Sands began by remarking that in the context of the global financial crisis of 2007–2008, governments were prepared to invest significant sums of money into preventing future financial crises. He posited that the investments made after the global financial crisis back then helped prevent an immediate financial crisis at the onset of the COVID-19 pandemic. Turning to the need for pandemic preparedness, Sands noted that it will require the level of funding being discussed by the G20 HLIP, but pointed out that the current global external funding for TB is only around $1 billion per year. This underinvestment in TB juxtaposed with the proposed amount of new funding for pandemic preparedness appears inequitable, with large sums of money designated to meet new and future threats that might kill people alongside hesitancy to spend much smaller amounts of money on diseases that are currently killing people. Even within high-TB-burden countries, funding is often not allocated equitably because the disease is primarily contracted by people outside of the elite class. Sands asked,

> How do we justify spending a lot of money on diseases that might kill people, when we are not spending remotely enough on diseases that are killing people right now? How do we lift both those boats simultaneously?

Tharman said in response that today's international financing of global health security—essentially composed of efforts to prevent and combat infectious disease threats—totals approximately $15 billion in governmental and philanthropic investments. At a minimum, an additional $15 billion is needed, one-third of which would be channeled through existing routes for specific missions, thereby significantly increasing funding for organizations. The remaining two-thirds could create a predictable, multilateral layer of funding to support the system by connecting silos. He stated that a central challenge is establishing governance of global health security that ensures attention is appropriately placed on areas of need and that financing is raised, rather than rediverted, for these areas. Tharman emphasized that the total funding needed pales in comparison to the costs of a major outbreak, thus the social return on these investments is high. Much synergy exists between addressing endemic diseases and preventing the next pandemic; therefore funding the former will strengthen the latter.

Amanda Glassman, executive vice president and senior fellow at the Center for Global Development and chief executive officer of the center's branch in Europe, asked about the finance implications and incentive opportunities regarding the TB burden in middle-income countries. She suggested that one reason only $1 billion in international financing has been directed at TB is because middle-income countries theoretically have the ability to independently finance these basic public health services. Tharman held that international financing support and incentives will be needed for investments in certain global public goods even for middle-income countries. Although low-income countries will require grant money, other forms of international financing can be effective for middle-income countries. He added that extending IFI support to middle-income countries for this defined purpose is in the world's interest.

Gail Cassell, senior lecturer on global health and social medicine at Harvard Medical School, asked how increased accountability and demonstrated, documented data can be used to show a return on investment (ROI). She also asked what body or governance structure might be best suited to reviewing accountability and ROI. Tharman suggested strengthening financial governance to raise substantially greater amounts of funds on a sustained basis. This need not require a cumbersome process involving a large number of country representatives. Instead, principles need to be clearly set along with rigor in their application. The G20 HLIP proposed achieving this through the formation of an expanded G20 grouping that also includes major developing regions, global health organizations, and major multilateral organizations. This group would be responsible for identifying gaps in the system, continuously assessing risks, and prioritizing funding needs. He added that the group would have a permanent secretariat. The actual deployment of funds would feature the commercial discipline involved in ensuring ROI—which, in this case, is a quantification of social returns on investment, rather than private returns. Collaboration between institutions would be encouraged to increase coordination on the ground. Tharman commented that sustaining high levels of funding from donors and the broader group of countries in the world will require good governance and demonstration that funds are being well used and achieving desired effects over time.

Cassell asked whether the G20 HLIP will continue to lead this effort. Tharman responded that HLIP has made a set of proposals that are currently being actively considered. Discussion continued during the United Nations (UN) General Assembly in September 2021 and in the G20 summit in October 2021. He hoped that concrete actions would be taken at the G20 summit to launch and strengthen these mechanisms over the next year. Sands called for capitalizing on the current opportunity to transform the approach to current and future health threats.

ACHIEVING SYNERGY IN GLOBAL HEALTH SECURITY PREPAREDNESS AGAINST RESPIRATORY PATHOGENS

Sands opened the panel discussion on achieving synergy in global health security preparedness against respiratory pathogens by suggesting that TB can either become a part of the pandemic preparedness agenda in making the world safer from future pathogens or it can be sidelined as a long-standing disease that primarily affects poor people, resulting in its deprioritization in the face of new threats. Sands asked for pragmatic next steps after the COVID-19 pandemic to prepare for future pandemics and to eliminate TB.

Large-Scale Vaccination Infrastructure

Presented by John Bell, Oxford University

Bell remarked that the COVID-19 pandemic has been a challenging time for global public health, in part because of the various silos rampant within the field. Infrastructure is needed that supports the capacity to address a wider range of pathogens, including both chronic pandemic pathogens (e.g., TB, malaria) and acute pandemic pathogens such as COVID-19. The current moment offers an opportunity to pivot from structures of the past to build a systematic program to prepare global public health for pathogen threats, both chronic and acute. The revolution in vaccines that has occurred during the COVID-19 pandemic began 15 years ago in an R&D agenda that was accelerated by the pandemic and has resulted in powerful, programmable platforms in the form of RNA and adenovirus. Additional candidate vaccines also show promise, including an adenovirus malaria vaccine for which data show nearly 80 percent efficacy (Yusuf et al., 2019) and the highly anticipated data on the M72 candidate vaccine for TB, Bell noted. Opportunities for multiplex coronavirus and influenza vaccines may become a cornerstone of future developments. The world's capacity to implement large-scale vaccination programs has been strengthened by expansion in vaccine manufacturing capacity (including RNA, adenovirus, and protein subunits) and the necessary supply chain of adjuvants. Such campaigns will not only address COVID-19 but also a host of other pathogens that could include TB. Maintaining the operability of facilities in interpandemic periods is important for pandemic preparedness, and the rollout of a set of potential adult vaccines would be an excellent method of facility maintenance, said Bell.

The capacity for low-income countries to implement large-scale vaccination programs remains limited, and absorption capacity will need to be substantially expanded to achieve near-universal COVID-19 vaccination coverage, Bell remarked. Information technology systems, logistics, and clinics are required to build a global public health system for adult vaccines. A strategy that expands capacity to administer vaccines for influenza, TB, malaria, and COVID-19 boosters would strengthen PPR efforts. Furthermore, additional injectables could be considered, such as long-acting, annual injectables for a variety of health needs (e.g., small interfering RNA for cardiometabolic disease protection, long-acting HIV drugs, or contraception). A system that prevents multiple diseases at once could generate massive efficiencies of scale, he added.

Another structure that could result from the COVID-19 pandemic is better genomic surveillance and sequencing associated with a global cloud infrastructure for managing data and providing immediate analysis, said Bell. Such a system could affect multiple major pathogens. Although it may be tempting to focus new systems on COVID-19, he cautioned against continuing to operate within silos. Instead, common infrastructure and systematic approaches can be created that address a range of different diseases while improving cost-effectiveness and ROI.

Identifying Alignments in Surveillance Efforts

Presented by Bruce Gellin, Rockefeller Foundation

Gellin echoed Bell's comments that using expanded vaccination capacity for vaccines beyond COVID-19 will aid in justifying the investments. For vaccines to be effective, they must turn into vaccinations. He suggested that the TB community can contribute its extensive experience in contact tracing, community-based surveillance, and community delivery. Seasonal and pandemic influenza, TB, and COVID-19 are all respiratory pathogens, thus maintaining silos for each pathogen is not the most effective approach to addressing these diseases.[4]

Bolstering early warning surveillance systems during interpandemic periods can improve detection capability and provide baseline data, said Gellin. Epidemiology, surveillance, and data sharing are currently being used to address COVID-19 variants. Although the process begins with genomic surveillance, the compilation of a range of data informs researchers of cur-

---

[4] Gellin added that when he worked on antimicrobial resistance, TB was in its own silo in spite of widespread awareness of MDR TB. He suggested that perhaps shifting language, for example, referring to extensively drug-resistant TB (XDR TB) as *variants* would garner more attention.

rent disease activity, areas where pathogens are emerging, and the degree to which outbreaks can be predicted. Gellin noted that the long history of TB can provide data for the surveillance system. The surveillance systems that have been created during the COVID-19 pandemic (e.g., the Rockefeller Foundation's Pandemic Prevention Institute, WHO's Hub for Pandemic and Epidemic Intelligence, the UK's Global Pandemic Radar) could productively collaborate like gears within an engine. Investments in early surveillance could enable targets to be established. Alignments between efforts would capitalize on the developments that stem from each pathogen, creating a common system for prevention, identification, surveillance, and treatment.

Applying Tuberculosis Research to the COVID-19 Pandemic
Presented by Rebecca Katz, Georgetown University

Katz described significant variation in TB mitigation approaches implemented across the United States and how this variation intersects with health security. In 2014, she conducted a study examining U.S. local-level capacity and policy around the use of isolation and quarantine as containment measures (Katz and Vaught, 2017). Interviews conducted with TB control officers around the United States informed case studies of TB outbreaks in the decade prior. The study's goal was to better understand the approaches used by local health departments to identify and contain outbreaks and to determine isolation protocols used. Katz described remarkable variation around the country in terms of (1) social distancing interventions, (2) handling of noncompliant patients by local public health entities, (3) the degree of judicial and community support, (4) financial resources, and (5) incentives and enablers used to maintain isolation of infectious TB patients. For instance, some jurisdictions placed infectious patients in negative pressure jail cells, while others enabled isolation by paying heating bills, delivering groceries, and providing electronic tablets and Wi-Fi to facilitate family communication. Identifying evidentiary standards, risk assessment, political will, and community support can inform how these factors affect the ability to institute social distancing policies. Katz noted that this study was informative of how jurisdictions later managed early COVID-19 cases. The purpose of the study was to use TB as a mechanism for understanding the capacity of health departments to implement physical distancing measures in a pandemic, and its findings demonstrate how capacity building for TB and PPR affect one another.

Katz and colleagues have mapped budgetary data for the Global Fund onto the joint external evaluation indicators of the International Health Regulations (Boyce et al., 2021). Although the Global Fund invested in TB—and not in pandemics—much of the TB work was pivoted to COVID-19.

Even prior to the pandemic, strengthened TB response and capacity building demonstrated direct links with health security capacity building. Examples of crossover capabilities include contact tracing and the ability to address antimicrobial resistance (AMR), which includes laboratory analysis and sequencing. Prior to the COVID-19 pandemic, the few examples of robust contact tracing efforts included sexually transmitted infections and TB tracing conducted in schools, airports, and among vulnerable populations, noted Katz. The Global Fund has used GeneXpert as a platform for both TB and COVID-19 in assessing overall laboratory capacity-building efforts and incentives, enablers, and enforcement of physical distancing measures for isolation and quarantine. Such overlaps indicate an opportunity for pragmatism in investments and strategies that consider how different programs affect one another, she added.

Innovation in Technology and Finance

Presented by Michael Callahan, Massachusetts General Hospital and United Therapeutics

Noting the destabilizing effects of TB upon public health infrastructures and all-cause failures, Callahan suggested that TB would be an appropriate addition to the global health security agenda. Operational public health intervention programs for TB have been decimated by a focus on COVID-19, whereas COVID-19 implementation strategies have benefited from therapy, surveillance, and other programs developed for TB. He likened this to the way in which PEPFAR work benefited the infrastructure, therapeutics delivery, and movement of samples in the response to the 2012–2013 Ebola outbreak in West Africa. Callahan suggested examining the destabilizing influences of a pandemic on the treatment of other diseases and assessing the ability to use preexisting infrastructure during a pandemic.

To justify the inclusion of TB in the global health security agenda from an evidentiary standpoint, Callahan highlighted data comparing the effects of TB and COVID-19. He shared that each year, 900,000 people die directly from TB disease, a figure that does not include secondary effects of long-term sequelae of highly toxic antimicrobials and infections from peripherally inserted central catheters for aminoglycoside treatment. While 4.7 million people died from COVID-19 within a 19-month period,[5] this rate will likely drop with continued distribution of quality vaccines, converting COVID-19 from a pandemic to an endemic. In contrast, he noted, TB has not reached endemicity thresholds despite the many years that humans have coexisted with

---

[5] Data as of September 16, 2021 from https://coronavirus.jhu.edu/data/mortality (accessed January 2, 2022).

the disease. Comparing the adjusted cost ratios of TB and COVID-19—without adjusting for age, gender, or comorbidities—underscores the high cost of treating TB. In his experience working in austere medical settings, treating MDR TB and XDR TB patients eliminates available capacity to treat other acute illnesses, including malaria and respiratory and diarrheal diseases. Callahan shared that the cost index accepted by WHO for MDR TB management in affluent nations is $152,000 and includes first-line therapy failures with isoniazid. In comparison, Kaiser Permanente calculated that the adjusted cost of hospital care for a COVID-19 patient in the United States and Canada—for cases not requiring extracorporeal membrane oxygenation or extended ventilation—ranges from $51,000 to $78,000 (Hackett, 2020).

Callahan highlighted innovations that could be used to address TB. New medical countermeasures include gene-encoded therapies and host modulating therapies. He underscored the challenges in acquiring funding for messenger RNA (mRNA) vaccines, noting that prior to the success of mRNA vaccines against COVID-19, 11 years elapsed before Moderna and BioNTech were funded by a second federal agency. He added that influenza vaccines are more technically challenging to develop, and these limits to the technology can only be expanded by rigorous competitive investment in multiple categories. To address TB, Callahan commented that from a strategic standpoint, the process of addressing *Mycobacterium tuberculosis* should focus on avoiding selection for resistance that will decimate antimicrobial classes used for other lifesaving therapeutic purposes, notably for respiratory infections. He mentioned the potential for host modulating therapies such as DNA therapies that can temporarily disrupt large encoded biologics and enzyme systems necessary for infection or target the bacteria itself. For example, there are phase 2 studies that have generated enthusiasm around the ability of host modulating therapies to deny a host enzyme system that is necessary to a pathogen for a short period of time, without exerting a selective pressure to lead to escape use. This area of inquiry is largely focused on retroviruses and drug-resistant hepatitis C viruses and is expanding into bacterial pathogens, including mycobacteria, he added.

Financial management is another area of innovation. The U.S. Agency for International Development's PREDICT program and the Defense Advanced Research Projects Agency (DARPA) have used financial management strategies that highlight diseases with low profit margins to capture the interest of foreign investors. Callahan remarked that a "twinning" strategy of coupling diseases with low profit margins to diseases with high net worth has been extraordinarily successful. For example, two hepatitis C drugs that generate $6 billion in annual revenue were yoked to drugs for dengue. This brought the dengue portfolio into phase 2 trials, but profit-seeking business interests abandoned it during licensing. Had DARPA held those drugs, better small-molecule inhibitors for dengue and other flaviviruses likely would have entered phase 3 studies and possibly even licensure to address a disease that infects over 400 million people each year.

This strategy may be useful for mycobacteria because several of the drug targets are conserved across other Gram-negative bacteria. Another strategy is using the target product profile for low- and middle-income countries (LMICs). Callahan commented that technologies to address HIV that did not work in cities such as Boston and London proved to be effective in directly inserted antiretroviral therapy programs in African countries. These less expensive, more effective therapies designed for LMIC settings were justified by their clinical usefulness and cost-effectiveness. The demonstrated value of these treatments then propelled their readoption by the high-income countries that made them and are now considered the standard of care. Moving forward, target product profiles should include the clinical treatment environment and the need for longitudinal patient monitoring, said Callahan. He added that treatment and release is now being used for a number of influenza therapies.

AMR and the selection of resistance should be reconciled with the clinical pragmatism of large-scale public health delivery systems, Callahan remarked. Antimicrobial stewardship programs in LMICs can be ineffective in the situation of an imminent, acute clinical decision to save a patient. He noted that devastating events have occurred when AMR was considered without understanding the rational use of antimicrobials for strategic reasons. For instance, if rifampicin is used as the empiric presumptive therapy for meningococcal disease to routinely treat thousands of children in sub-Saharan Africa, subsequent cases of TB in the region will be rifampicin-resistant in the following months to years, said Callahan. Thus, understanding the bystander public health casualties is important when addressing AMR.

Discussion

Surveillance Systems

A participant asked about the features a system would need to boost national capacity for pandemic preparedness surveillance while simultaneously benefiting people with TB symptoms presenting at primary health care clinics. Gellin emphasized that surveillance is more than remote data aggregation and must include local capacity for identification and analysis. The COVID-19 pandemic has developed the recognition that localities and central focus points alike need to understand both the big picture and the specific on-the-ground implications. Data sharing also plays a role: the sourcing, sharing, and use of data at all levels contribute to an effective system. However, data sharing is built upon trust. Katz remarked that strengthening the health care system overall affects surveillance. Improved access to care worldwide increases the likelihood a person will be seen by a medical professional, have their symptoms diagnosed, and obtain lab results. Thus, building a strong health care system can simultaneously strengthen pandemic preparedness and address population health concerns. The entire public health and health care system—rather than a specific disease—should be considered in determining the systems to build.

Tracking Progress in Prevention

Sands remarked that among the attractions of disease-specific silos are the advantages of easily defined outcomes and highly focused targets. For example, desired outcomes of a TB-specific program include decreases in infections and deaths. Measuring performance becomes more difficult for a system focused on multiple pathogens, sustainable capability, and integration. He noted that results of health systems investments that were not directly linked to disease-specific outcomes have been mixed, and asked how a system can be highly focused without using silos and managing performance while achieving integration. Katz replied that the activities that are measured become the activities that are performed. However, the health security and pandemic preparedness space has never been measured well. Before the COVID-19 pandemic, it was difficult to raise sufficient funds to build PPR capacity owing to the lack of a compelling metric (e.g., a measure for how much safer the population would be). In contrast, TB and malaria programs are able to generate figures on the numbers of lives saved. Katz suggested developing a new approach to formulating ROI to determine what types of PPR investments are needed and how these are tracked.

Bell recounted that approximately 20 years ago he met someone at a workshop who had obtained a large amount of funding for global TB control. When he asked how this had been managed, the person replied that he was ruthless in communicating the terrible aspects of TB while dismissing all other diseases. Bell suggested this reflected a culture in which researchers interested in broad, systems-based interventions cannot obtain funding, but this culture appears to have changed in the modern day. A potential strategy is to develop a system that focuses on surveillance and vaccination for a single pathogen, then expand it to additional pathogens once the system is established. Bell emphasized the importance of developing measurable outcomes and the effect of efficiencies of scale on ROIs.

Diagnostics Technology

Kenneth Castro, professor of global health and epidemiology at Emory University, stated that in some countries with low TB incidence—including the Netherlands and the United States—universal genotyping is used to better understand transmission dynamics and to identify locations warranting additional attention. He remarked that investment in laboratory services infrastructure and rapid feedback capacity should include TB and other infectious pathogens. Gellin echoed the importance of establishing broader surveillance. Creating a surveillance system begins with collecting and examining samples, and genomic surveillance could become the standard moving forward. The opportunity to develop simpler at-home diagnostics could also play a role by empowering people to better understand their risks when going out in public. Offering incentives is a potential strategy for developing such technologies for TB and a range of respiratory pathogens, he added.

Cassell remarked that new technology is being developed for COVID-19 that enables at-home diagnostic and screening stations to perform tests in the field instead of relying on laboratories—potentially reducing both expense and personnel required for testing as well—and emphasized how important a point-of-care diagnostic could be in addressing TB. She asked about other examples of progress and how these may affect technological advances for TB. Callahan replied that the international community has focused on lateral flow assays for muramyl dipeptide and other TB markers. Current challenges relate to technical complications in obtaining sputum samples and preparing them for the tests. Groups including Wellcome Trust, the Tropical Diseases Research Centre, and the Agency for Science, Technology and Research (A*STAR) Singapore have been working on sample preparation technology that could revolutionize TB diagnostics. For example, A*STAR is working to address TB risk in Singapore by controlling TB in other nations; it has invested in a program for the diagnosis of any lower respiratory tract infection that has expansive usefulness outside of TB. Gellin highlighted the need for diagnostic technology that can be moved distally, but he cautioned that when using at-home and in-field testing, efforts should be made to capture the data to avoid losing it for the public health surveillance system.

Factors Affecting the Perception of Urgency

Sands remarked on the sense of urgency around COVID-19 that is lacking with respect to TB, posing challenges to mobilizing political will and scientific interest in the disease. He presented a scenario in which a new disease emerges that kills 1 million people a year, has a latent infection rate of 25 percent of the world, and creates variants that evolve in ways that make it extremely difficult to treat, and carry high case fatality rates. In such a scenario, would a vaccine timeline of 4 to 5 years suffice, or would the 100-day target apply?[6] Would the pace at which accurate point-of-care

---

[6] The 100-day target has been discussed as a goal for PPR in a number of initiatives including the American Pandemic Preparedness Plan and the pandemic preparedness partnership of the G7 (see https://assets.publishing.service.gov.uk/government/uploads/system/uploads/attachment_data/file/992762/100_Days_Mission_to_respond_to_future_pandemic_threats__3_.pdf, accessed January 2, 2022).

diagnostics are being developed be considered satisfactory? Sands suggested that the length of time TB has existed has engendered a familiarity with the disease that undermines the sense of urgency that would arise if it were a novel disease with identical consequences.

Callahan believes that a new disease with the same morbidity, mortality, and economic effects as TB would generate a startled response, in contrast to the apparent fatigue around TB. New arguments for combating TB are economic and financial, and rebalancing within the global coalition from public health government to corporate and civic bodies is taking place, he noted. For example, an Islamic health coalition associated with the Red Crescent is focusing efforts on TB throughout Indonesia in response to the devastation TB has caused in mosques and rural communities, as well as the complexity of accessing care deemed "halal"—or permissible—by the Imam. Callahan suggested that capturing the attention of coalitions that are not traditional public health groups could energize the effort because these coalitions bring new targets for measurement and are able to see that TB causes business disruption, economic devastation, and bystander casualties involving other diseases.

Currently, governments and populations in all parts of the world are determining the "tolerable" rates of COVID-19 as calculations are made regarding policy decisions, reopening schools, investment levels, and measures that are recommended or required, said Katz. She remarked on the subjective nature of tolerance as it pertains to rates of infection, morbidity, and mortality. Personal calculations will not necessarily match those of political leaders, while the calculations of political leaders vary in different parts of the world. She suggested that the current awareness of COVID-19 morbidity and mortality presents an opportunity to recast conversations about diseases that the public has normalized. Sands added that normalization is a human coping mechanism that can lead to accepting things that should be deemed unacceptable. Gellin remarked that the conversations around learning to manage COVID-19 in the event it cannot be eradicated would be a challenge should the same thinking be applied to TB. Owing to the long-standing nature of TB and its lack of visibility among populations that are not contracting the disease, people may be complacent about addressing it. Should that prove to be the case, the TB community will need to improve efforts to raise awareness regarding the numbers of people affected by this disease, stated Gellin. Bell noted that although the public tolerates seasonal influenza that kills tens of thousands of people in the United States each year, alarm arises when there is a pandemic or epidemic, leading to greater attention to vaccines. The way in which people address these issues is not always logical, as reflected in the management of TB.

Sands noted that people tend to be more willing to tolerate diseases that are not killing people in their close circles, and less troubled about a disease that causes deaths in other parts of the world or even in other parts of the city. This has been the case with TB and HIV, which disproportionally affect marginalized and poor populations. Unless PPR efforts address this tendency to normalize a level of risk to certain parts of society, it may translate to a high level of ongoing threat with high morbidity and mortality cost, he warned, predicting that the tendency to be complacent about high levels of mortality in poorer or marginalized populations will continue until it is disrupted. Bell added that the issues that directly affect people's lives are the ones that spur them to take action. Gellin noted a similarity in complacency around climate change. Although the effects of climate change seem to be becoming more evident to the public, the lack of direct implications on people's lives thus far has resulted in a lack of urgency. Katz commented that a benefit among the terrible aspects of the COVID-19 pandemic is an increase in global population awareness of disease communicability.

Using the energy and perspectives of communities that have traditionally been outside of the health system could bring in new ideas and increase levels of commitment to addressing TB, said Sands. He recounted a quote attributed to medical anthropologist Paul Farmer, "The idea that some lives matter less is the root of all that's wrong with the world." Sands suggested that a PPR agenda that marginalizes the TB response would not fulfill an inclusive vision of protecting everyone. Bell replied that this is even more the case with malaria, which tends to be less prevalent than TB in Western countries. This raises issues around how pandemics are defined and who defines them, said Sands. Common usage of the term *pandemic* seems to refer to the disease death rates in wealthy countries, and this perception should be addressed in PPR efforts.

Capitalizing on the COVID-19 Pandemic

Sands asked the panelists to offer final thoughts on the role of TB in the PPR agenda. Bell described a scenario that could take place over the course of the next 18–24 months, in which COVID-19 becomes broadly controlled in developed economies. At that point, interest in PPR declines, marking a return to the status quo without advancing efforts to fight TB. To avoid this scenario, he suggested capitalizing on the current sense of urgency by putting structures in place for PPR from which TB efforts would benefit. Bell added that it will likely be several decades before another such opportunity to create PPR systems appears. Gellin said that instead of focusing efforts on one disease and hoping these efforts will benefit other diseases, lessons learned from multiple diseases should be packaged together and can be addressed synergistically. Bell added that this approach creates a multiplier for results and thus a more persuasive argument for investments.

Katz was hopeful that the panic-to-neglect cycle will last longer than 2 years before returning to a phase of neglect, but how long the world's attention on PPR will be sustained is uncertain. Should the strategy developed by the G20 HLIP prove successful in raising billions of dollars annually for PPR, this would capitalize on the current opportunity to make smart investments in a holistic, global system that better addresses all biological threats. Callahan commented that there is cause for optimism in the potentially transformative innovations occurring in new medical countermeasures, lateral flow assays, point-of-care diagnostics for TB, and sample prep technology. In the past, some promising technologies have been stymied and suppressed within the legacy disease environment, but the dated system for TB could be restructured to be innovative and capitalize on technological advances. Sands predicted that including TB in the PPR agenda would scale opportunity, but TB's inclusion will require bringing to bear the efforts of leaders, policy makers, and the TB advocacy community. The history of TB demonstrates that fully addressing the disease will not happen by its own accord, he added.

MAKING THE CASE FOR FINANCING TUBERCULOSIS ELIMINATION

Margaret Hamburg, interim vice president of Global Biological Policy and Programs for the Nuclear Threat Initiative, moderated the panel on the financing of programs and implementation of policies directed at the ultimate goal of TB elimination. In terms of a panic-to-neglect cycle, current public awareness of the threat of communicable diseases and the magnitude of health tragedies—and social and economic dislocations—they can cause provides an opportunity for action. At the same time, an environment of fatigue from COVID-19 can present challenges to a public overwhelmed by living in a world of biological threats. Furthermore, as the world emerges from the current COVID-19 crisis, many priorities will compete for attention and funding. Investments in TB elimination simultaneously address health, humanitarian, and safety needs.

Economic Analysis of the Cost of Failing to Achieve the End TB Targets

Presented by Mike Reid, University of California, San Francisco

Reid outlined the full-income cost of failing to end the TB epidemic. The Lancet Commission TB strategy calls for a 90 percent reduction of the 2015 TB deaths by the year 2030 (Reid et al., 2019). He remarked that meeting this target seems highly improbable, and that the 2019 report highlighted that achieving this target by 2045 is also unlikely. In the context of the

COVID-19 pandemic, it is critical for high-TB-burden countries and their donor partners to understand why ending TB is essential.

Unfortunately, the overall evidence on the economics of TB has been heterogeneous and has lacked a comprehensive assessment of TB epidemics' effects on economic welfare, said Reid. Numerous studies have used a variety of tools to assess the economic effect of TB, including the macroeconomic implications of TB treatment and control activities. Commissioned by the Global TB Caucus in 2017, KPMG conducted an analysis on the effect of TB mortality on per capita domestic groups by projecting estimated economic losses attributable to TB-related mortality between 2015 and 2030 (Global TB Caucus, 2017). The analysis found that maintaining the TB status quo and failing to achieve the UN Sustainable Development Goals (SDGs) would result in 28 million TB deaths within that 15-year time, at a global economic cost of nearly $1 trillion. The greatest losses in GDP were projected for Southeast Asia. Reid added that such macroeconomic studies that measure the effect of health improvements on economic productivity do not necessarily capture the intrinsic value that people place on their improved health. For this reason, many economists have asserted the usefulness of a full-income approach to assessing the effect of investing in health.

A full-income approach accounts for the value of additional life years in assessing economic productivity (Jamison et al., 2013). Reid described how two countries may have identical GDP but have starkly different TB burdens. The population of the country with low TB burden, "country A," lives longer and in better health than the population of "country B," where more people die from TB. An approach using GDP as the only measure of health does not capture the monetary value of country A's better performance. National income accounts do not reflect the reduced mortality risk in country A. In contrast, a full-income approach seeks to capture the value of life years gained by including the value of change in annual mortality rates in assessing changes in GDP. Reid remarked that estimating the growth of a country's full income—rather than using GDP alone—provides a more accurate, complete picture of the value of investments.

Reid and colleagues evaluated the effect of investing in TB programs and the economic dividend that could be generated from reduced TB mortality (Silva et al., 2021). The analysis involved calculations of life expectancy gains from 2020 to 2050 under three scenarios in 120 countries. The first scenario featured the steady 2 percent decline in TB deaths that signifies business as usual. The second scenario envisioned meeting the SDG target of ending the TB epidemic by 2030; the third scenario involved meeting the target by 2045. Additionally, the researchers attempted to evaluate the excess deaths caused by disruptions in TB services related to the COVID-19 pandemic. Reid noted that this evaluation involved assumptions and outputs from a modeling paper commissioned by the Stop TB Partnership (Cilloni et al., 2020).

Researchers determined the current full-income loss associated with TB using 2018 data, in which approximately 1.4 million people died from all forms of TB. The full-income losses were estimated to be $580 billion, or approximately $407,000 per TB death. The highest losses were concentrated in sub-Saharan Africa, a region that accounted for $200 billion in accrued losses. In other words, had the 1.4 million TB deaths in 2018 been averted, $580 billion of full-income losses would also have been averted, Reid explained. Additionally, life expectancy at birth for individuals living in those 120 countries would increase by an average of 0.47 years.

The analysis estimated that should the current 2 percent rate of declining TB deaths continue annually until 2050, 32 million deaths will occur, said Reid. The economic losses caused by these deaths are estimated to be $17.5 trillion. Southeast Asia would experience the highest economic losses—totaling approximately $7 trillion—and countries in sub-Saharan Africa would see the greatest effect on life expectancy with a reduction of 0.84 years. In contrast, meeting the SDG target by 2030 would result in an estimated 8 million deaths over the next decade and an associated economic loss of $4 trillion dollars. Meeting the SDG target by 2045 would avert an estimated 13.7 million deaths and $7.3 trillion in economic losses. Therefore, the overall cost of inadequate action incurred by meeting the SDG target in 2045 rather than in 2030 is over $3.3 trillion and 5.7 million deaths, Reid noted.

Reid and his colleagues also assessed the effect of COVID-19 on TB-related economic losses by estimating the health care costs resulting from excess TB deaths in three countries (Reid et al., 2020). They found that TB cases were likely to increase as a result of COVID-19-related service disruptions in 2020. A 3-month suspension of programs during lockdown and a 10-month recovery period for programs to return to prepandemic activity were estimated to result in an excess of TB-related health costs totaling $1.95 billion in India, $96 million in Ukraine, and $29 million in Kenya. Applying the full-income approach to these modeling assumptions, researchers estimated that even in the best-case scenario of the SDG target being met in 2030, the COVID-19-related disruptions in TB services in 2020 could create $447 billion in full-income losses (Silva et al., 2021). Reid stated that even the relatively short-lived disruption of TB services caused by the COVID-19 pandemic is predicted to lead to substantial full-income losses in the next 15 years.

Outlining the limitations of the analysis, Reid noted that the full-income analysis did not capture the economic implications of nonfatal TB. Additionally, the estimates of TB mortality are crude and may be conservative, which affects the economic estimates based on these figures. However, the research indicates that substantial full-income losses will arise if efforts to respond to the TB epidemic are not increased. Moreover, the amounts of funding currently being invested in TB programs pale in comparison to the huge potential economic losses. He added that these findings have important implications for ministries of finance and donor partners.

The research provides compelling reasons for investing in the scale-up of evidence-based, patient-centered programs, including increased focus on high-burden settings, in concert with a broader global health security agenda. It also provides evidence in support of greater prioritization of investment in health by high-burden countries, said Reid. Governments can be incentivized to increase efforts, especially given that the benefits of investment are estimated to exceed the cost by a factor of five (Reid et al., 2019). Furthermore, these investments strengthen global public goods from which all nations will benefit. Reid asserted that the current moment affords a propitious, unique opportunity to use the political will and investment in responding to COVID-19 and preventing future pandemics toward efforts to end TB. COVID-19 and TB serve as reminders of the value of prioritizing health, allocating financial and human resources for universal health coverage, and addressing the needs of vulnerable populations in particular.

Making a Compelling Case for Strengthening TB Control and the Consequences Thereof

Presented by Bjorn Lomborg, Copenhagen Consensus Center

Lomborg explained that his work involves examining a vast range of areas to determine where the application of resources may be most effective. Working with more than 300 of the world's top economists, including Nobel laureates, the Copenhagen Consensus Center (CCC) explores issues such as climate, health, and HIV in countries including Haiti, Bangladesh, India, Ghana, Malawi, and Uganda. CCC has analyzed the SDGs in an effort to prioritize them. The SDGs include approximately 300 targets, many of which are not currently on track to be met by 2030. Lomborg noted that the CCC worked with over 100 economists to prepare publications on a large range of topics in order to evaluate the costs and benefits of the SDG areas, partnered with media outlets in 20 low-income countries to publicize the research; the CCC also published a large book with Cambridge University Press and a shorter book for increased accessibility that details the research findings (Lomborg, 2015, 2018). Lastly, CCC created a one-page synopsis that lists the cost and benefit analyses for 80 different activities within the SDG agenda.[7]

The analysis identified decreasing TB deaths as a good investment, with every dollar spent on TB prevention and treatment generating $43 worth of

---

[7] The synopsis is available from https://www.copenhagenconsensus.com/sites/default/files/post2015brochure_m.pdf (accessed December 15, 2021).

social good, said Lomborg. The costs of addressing TB include $4.3 billion for latent TB screening to identify the estimated 2.7 million undiagnosed cases each year, $2.2 billion for treatment of 5.8 million people with drug-sensitive TB, and $1.6 billion for the 500,000 people with MDR TB. This totals $8.1 billion in annual spending—or $907 per person with TB—to address all TB cases worldwide. Savings in life years was used as the defining benefit of these interventions in this analysis, which is estimated at an average savings of 20 life years. Researchers used the disability-adjusted life year (DALY) metric to measure the overall disease burden of early TB-related death and used time discounting to account for loss of future healthy years of life. Calculations were conducted with different discount rates and DALY benefit amounts to account for a variety of backgrounds. The analysis used 3 and 5 percent discount rates and DALY benefit amounts of $1,000 and $5,000. The median benefit of this range of calculations is $38,594. Factoring in the cost of $907 per person with TB, the resulting benefit-to-cost ratio is 43. This signifies that $43 of social good will be generated from each dollar spent on eliminating TB, Lomborg explained.

A high benefit-to-cost ratio can influence decision makers in investment choices, and CCC has found that tackling TB is one of the fundamentally best investments that can be made for many countries, said Lomborg. As part of its work in India, the organization partnered with Tata Trusts to form Rajasthan Priorities.[8] The group determined that TB—which kills about 40,000 people in Rajasthan each year—was the most effective use of investment dollars. Sixty percent of Rajasthani people with TB receive treatment in private care settings, but it is often substandard. Although some may argue that the solution is moving TB care to the public sphere, Lomborg noted that the most realistic solution is to improve private care. The national strategic plan supported by Prime Minister Modi focuses on engagement with private care providers by offering subsidies for people to receive high-quality diagnostic tests and TB treatment in both private and public provider settings. The plan also offers patients treatment adherence support through call centers and works with private care settings to improve TB notification practices. Lomborg noted that the average annual cost for the services included in the plan is $2 million, but the benefit is $373 million. In this case, the benefit-to-cost ratio is 171, meaning that if you spend one dollar, it can deliver up to 171 dollars of social benefit derived from the program. He emphasized how influential the benefit-to-cost ratio can be in establishing TB as one of the best investments a country can make.

---

[8] This group engaged with stakeholders from the Rajasthani government, academic institutions, and the private sector. Bibek Debroy, chairman of the Economic Advisory Council to Prime Minister Modi, was an eminent Rajasthan Priorities panelist. See https://www.copenhagenconsensus.com/rajasthan-priorities.

CCC's current project, Halftime for the SDGs, is assessing how much progress has been made on SDGs by 2022. Although the SDGs are approaching the halfway point on the timeline, the world is not on track to make most or possibly any of the promises made by 2030. Given that reality, the Halftime for the SDGs project is highlighting 15 goals determined to be the smartest investments for the global community to focus on, and TB is one of the best investments among the SDGs, said Lomborg. CCC will be working with other organizations, such as Stop TB, to advocate for the prioritization of TB and other top investments with decision makers.

Smart Investments in Ending TB

Presented by Mark Dybul, Georgetown University

Dybul highlighted the effect of COVID-19 on TB interventions, noting that India—a country that had been increasing TB investment, as Lomborg described—has substantially reduced investment in TB over the past 12–18 months because of the pandemic. He added that in the current environment, persuasive ROI arguments for individual interventions are making direct links to PPR. Despite being in the second year of the COVID-19 pandemic, a global response to the pandemic has yet to develop; this was the focus of the G20 summit in October 2021. Nationalism has impeded progress on a global plan to address a pandemic that affects everyone, including wealthy people and high-income nations, he added. This challenging atmosphere makes it more difficult to address a disease such as TB that affects marginalized people in lower-income countries.

Dybul said that for TB interventions to be effective in the current context, they should be linked to pandemics, both in terms of determining the steps that are needed now and in anticipating needs 5 to 10 years in the future. Moreover, this discussion of needs must translate into action; then, the systems created must also be sustained. He remarked that the best way to sustain PPR systems is to intentionally invest in current existing pandemics, such as TB, rather than focusing on interpandemics. Systems built for current pandemics can then be used for surge capacity when intervening pandemics, such as COVID-19, arise. Investing in systems for TB has revealed that a strong ground game is the most effective approach. This involves identifying cases in areas where people may be resistant to health care and health systems and conducting contact tracing. The process also requires diagnostics, particularly molecular diagnostics (e.g., GeneXpert platform pivoted from TB diagnostics to testing for COVID-19 in low-income countries). Once cases are identified, a system should be in place to provide treatment to people who may lack access to health care or be resistant to the health care system. Dybul emphasized that the components of such a system are simultaneously high-return investments for TB and high-return investments for sustainable PPR capability.

Many people who contract TB are marginalized and do not generally access health systems, said Dybul. A number of current TB programs are successful in finding people with the disease, providing care services, and conducting contact tracing in low-income settings. Advances in diagnostics and molecular diagnostics present an opportunity to build TB systems that expand beyond response to include surveillance and preparedness. The Stop TB Partnership has focused on mobile diagnostics, and these could include TB as well as diabetes, hypertension, breast cancer, prostate cancer, and other diseases. Mobile units could have magnetic resonance imaging and X-ray machines. Not only is such a system necessary to address TB, it also provides primary health care, noted Dybul. Momentum is growing toward strengthening primary health care, which is itself a PPR system component. He remarked that the types of TB interventions Reid and Lomborg discussed are precisely the systems needed for primary health care and PPR. Placing TB in the context of building and sustaining preparedness and response systems before the next pandemic creates a persuasive argument for investment in the current environment.

Implications for Tuberculosis from the High-Level Independent Panel on Financing the Global Commons for Pandemic Preparedness and Response

Amanda Glassman, Center for Global Development

Glassman said that the G20 HLIP has examined the economic rationale for financing PPR and the role of subsidies at the international level, otherwise known as international financing. HLIP distinguished international financing from aid based on their purposes, and determined that international financing should be reserved for global public goods. A global public good is a good or activity that is nonexclusionary at the global or regional level, meaning that the benefits of its consumption accrue beyond an individual, a local government, or a nation. These goods are often not provided by the market, and they tend to lack a political constituency, because the benefits of prevention are intangible and not immediately visible.

Global public goods include the development of a vaccine that prevents transmission of an infectious disease, said Glassman. Considered a "best shot public good," a single nation or even an individual can develop a vaccine that will benefit everyone if used. Another type of public good is known as a "weakest link public good." For example, an individual country's poor performance in controlling an infectious disease such as TB can drive adverse outcomes beyond its borders. Infectious disease control is therefore a "weakest link good" where the actions at the weakest link in the chain affect the entire world's outcomes. Glassman remarked that HLIP has argued that international financing—not aid—should create clear incentives for governments around the world to devote more resources to these uses. Some governments require international subsidies before they are able to devote resources to these goods, because the competing demands on scarce public spending are relatively so substantial that they often lead to underprioritization of public goods. For example, many low-income countries spend a larger percentage of their budgets on hospital care than on preventative primary health care.

HLIP acknowledged that investments in the broad set of actions needed to combat both existing and emerging infectious diseases are a contribution to global public goods, said Glassman. Initiatives addressing TB care, poverty, housing, and cash transfers could influence the trajectory of TB and of health systems overall. Controlling an infectious disease involves health care coverage, access to care, hospital availability, workforce, quality care, coverage of specific interventions, community engagement, health behaviors, and innovation and technology for medical countermeasures. HLIP has proposed three strategies to address an area of great need in which numerous existing organizations are already working:

1. Push complementary financing to existing entities already working in this space (e.g., WHO, CEPI, Gavi, the Global Fund) to enable scaling up of efforts.
2. Focus on high priority—but relatively underaddressed—global public goods that are currently inadequately funded or are funded in a piecemeal or irrational fashion (e.g., surveillance of respiratory pathogens, end-to-end financing of medical countermeasures from R&D to procurement).
3. Create financial incentives for countries to increase preparedness across the board.

Glassman outlined how these strategies apply to TB. Although the disease has existed for at least 9,000 years and economic development has helped to address it, MDR TB is a cross-border threat that signifies a "global public bad" that must be constrained. The core agenda for existing funding is expanding screening and first-line treatment using high-quality medicines, ensuring adherence, and enhancing progress on surveillance. Glassman noted that exploration of how to accelerate progress or make more effective use of funds does not discount the efforts of the numerous organizations working in this space. The first HLIP strategy could enable scaling up of these current efforts. Regarding surveillance, although the Global Fund invests in surveillance efforts, significant challenges to quality persist. These include difficulty in conducting continuous surveillance of drug resistance, limited understanding of in-country geographic distribution of drug resistance, limited capacity to detect outbreaks or hotspots, and limited engagement of private providers. Glassman suggested that the pandemic preparedness effort focus on improving surveillance, potentially by combining surveillance of TB with that of other pathogens.

She noted that accepting government self-reports on their coverage of screening and treatment raises issues for the current TB response. Academic literature indicates a discrepancy between self-reports and researchers' observations in terms of growth of MDR TB or stagnant or increasing TB case rates. A thorough understanding of the circumstances cannot be gleaned in the absence of an adequate surveillance system. Additional funding could help define a quality surveillance system to address respiratory pathogens overall, including TB, influenza, and COVID-19. This system could then be measured in terms of completeness, accuracy, and timeliness, and these data would ideally be in the public domain, said Glassman.

Significant TB burden exists within middle-income countries that have the capacity to fully fund excellent TB programs, Glassman stated. However, competing demands for care, which have been exacerbated by COVID-19, hinder the full funding of TB efforts. Furthermore, TB primarily affects low-income communities within these countries where people may wait to seek care until later in their disease trajectories. The political economy of prevention complicates screening; people who are very poor will tend not to use preventative care services because of the substantial opportunity cost involved. This issue is often not addressed when developing programs, she noted.

Additionally, governments tend to opt for purchasing low-quality medicine because of the decreased cost, despite the availability of higher-quality medicine through the Global Fund's pooled procurement facilities. She suggested that new funding should act in cooperation with existing funding to include incentives for using high-quality medicine. Historically, small grants have been issued to civil society to provide service among key populations. However, population-based public health projects are insufficient to meet the need, said Glassman. Multilateral development banks could be used during this economic crisis to incentivize increases in budgeted spending for this purpose, surveillance performance, and the use of pooled procurement mechanisms. Financing mechanisms for R&D that engage middle-income country purchasers could also encourage innovation. For example, advanced market commitments could illustrate the savings that a country such as India could expect via investing in these innovations. Glassman remarked on the opportunity to find synergies with PPR that address both old and new pandemics.

Discussion

Engaging Political Leadership

Hamburg stated that despite the remarkable ROI of treating TB, the level of disease burden, and the numerous consequences of the disease, efforts to eliminate TB have been underfunded and underappreciated for many decades. This underscores the importance of engaging ministers of both finance and health in TB elimination efforts.[9] Hamburg asked how information regarding the reality of TB can be used to engage critical decision makers, such as foreign ministers, in moving TB efforts forward. Lomborg pointed out that if there were a simple answer, TB would have been fully addressed by now. TB, along with many other underfunded items on the global agenda, does not tend to attract people's attention. In the case of HIV, fear that the spread of disease could escalate out of control swayed many decision makers. In contrast, TB has existed for a long time and does not appear to be escalating: many people continue to die from it, yet it does not cause alarm. To address this tragic lack of urgency in the face of TB death rates, he suggested helping finance ministers understand that TB spending is a good investment that is not about getting things right but is about getting them less wrong.

Dybul echoed the importance of engaging finance members, noting that once India's finance minister and prime minister became involved, the country's TB efforts began to increase. This in turn garnered the attention of chief executive officers, such as those in Rajasthan. Movement on this issue requires engagement from political leadership, but gaining buy-in from finance ministers is challenging, because many people who die from TB are poor, marginalized, and do not tend to go to hospitals. Dybul noted that India and countries in Southeast Asia with high TB burdens are not low-income countries, but they have many competing priorities and treating TB in poor, marginalized populations will not boost the economy in the way that other investments might. However, COVID-19 has highlighted how quickly a pathogen can spread in urban centers. This heightened awareness offers an opportunity to engage with policy makers and emphasize that responding to existing pandemics will build and sustain systems needed for the next new pandemic.

Dybul noted that the diagnostic systems and approaches needed to address TB are relevant to other respiratory diseases and can be incorporated into the PPR system, thus the current moment also presents an opportunity to

---

[9] She noted in the case of HIV, once finance and military leaders understood the ramifications of the disease in domains beyond health, HIV was addressed in a serious and sustained fashion.

highlight how investments made now in TB and PPR systems could result in tremendous future savings. Reid added that COVID-19 has highlighted the economic dividend of investing in health more generally, providing a context for investing in TB specifically. Additionally, the HIV response demonstrated that civil society can influence governments by voicing discontent with mortality rates. The TB community could do more to empower civil society voices in high-burden countries to apply pressure to governmental leaders, he added.

Targeted Versus Systemwide Interventions for Tuberculosis

Hamburg noted that the creation of silos within global health may have inadvertently decreased the broad value of investments and missed opportunities for synergy. She highlighted Lomborg's argument that all SDGs cannot be met by 2030, and that therefore some of them should be prioritized. She asked Lomborg whether these ideas conflict with one another or if synergies and system strengthening can be pursued within the context of TB, given that advancing R&D, improving public health and disease control, and creating health systems that are better able to manage patients will also increase preparation for other respiratory diseases and threats. Lomborg replied that this is a methodological issue. Addressing one silo at a time is simpler than looking across a range of areas, because most data pertain to individual silos. Additionally, an argument made for a specific threat can be more effective than one for a broad range of needs. Furthermore, systems that cut across silos may include highly effective programs as well as noneffective pieces, in which case the overall effect of the effort may be diluted, said Lomborg.

Glassman suggested that the COVID-19 pandemic could serve as a powerful motivator to invest in surveillance that would benefit TB efforts. For instance, at the start of the COVID-19 pandemic, India received negative attention when it was unable to conduct accurate death counts, even in the country's capital. Given the possibility of a future influenza pandemic, creating a system that can use the same equipment, techniques, and metrics to address multiple respiratory pathogens could prove helpful on a number of fronts. Additionally, existing disease burdens can be used to assess the accuracy of surveillance systems. For example, data from serosurveys can be compared to health services data to identify areas of improvement for health services data collection. Glassman remarked that TB efforts and cross-silo systems need not be juxtaposed, as both can benefit from joint investments and the current political climate in response to COVID-19.

Closing Reflections

Hamburg asked the panelists for final comments. Reid remarked on the need for a global health framework that prioritizes the integration of universal health care and the health security agenda; TB provides a context for developing such a framework and should be prioritized. Lomborg commented that in an environment of competing priorities, TB should be repeatedly emphasized as an excellent investment to gain buy-in from heads of state and finance ministers. Dybul noted that in spite of the COVID-19 Delta variant, there is persistent nationalism around COVID-19 and a failure to understand that variants can develop and cross borders. He stated that the likelihood of a vaccine-resistant variant is high, and that it is not yet known whether the Mu or Lambda variants will resist vaccines. It is possible that COVID-19 will become endemic in lower-income countries, like TB and malaria, while other regions largely ignore the threat as soon as the crisis has passed in their areas. Now is the time to disrupt this long-standing pattern by building the capacities for protection through a global systemwide response.

Glassman emphasized the importance of checks and balances in designing systems to address pathogens. Many mechanisms solely fund governments—with a resultant lack of transparency—but complementary investment can fund universities, civil society, and research institutes in responding to TB, COVID-19, and other pathogens. She added that some governments will never prioritize response efforts, so the global health community should develop techniques to raise awareness and increase the political costs associated with failing to finance a response. Furthermore, communities working on existing diseases should view the health security agenda as an opportunity rather than as competition, she said. Advocacy should focus on replenishing global funding for Gavi and generating funds to forge connections and address the gaps highlighted by workshop participants. Hamburg remarked that a powerful case can be made to create needed systems, but advocates must make this case to the appropriate policy makers for those ideas to translate into sustained action backed by political will and commitment.

FINAL COMMENTS

In her final comments on the workshop, Cassell remarked that of all the innovations needed to address TB, diagnostics are prime. Better diagnostics are required both to identify infected patients and to generate data that illustrate the level of need regarding TB. A UN meeting was held in 2000 to determine efforts for the eight Millennium Development Goals (MDG). Noting that the sixth MDG was "to combat HIV/AIDS, malaria, and other diseases"—and that TB was one of the "other diseases"—Cassell suggested that this workshop has provided rationale for rephrasing the goal as combating "TB and other diseases." Ministers of finance and health can be powerful advocates for investing in systems to address TB. Often the situation is framed as requiring a policy solution, when in actuality it is an action solution that is needed, said Cassell. She echoed Callahan's comments regarding the need to create actionable priorities and to advocate for these with heads of state, finance ministers, and health ministers.

Recounting National Academy of Medicine meetings organized with the Russian Medical Academy and with National Academies in China to address MDR TB (IOM, 2011, 2014), Cassell wondered about the potential role that the U.S. National Academy of Sciences might take in developing and advocating for actionable priorities. From her position on the steering committee of the InterAcademy Partnership for Science, Health, and Policy, Hamburg believes that the organization would welcome the chance to use its network of academies and regional associations of academies in identifying key priorities for action and in engaging their scientific, public health, and medical communities in this effort.[10] Furthermore, Hamburg remarked that engaging the full range of stakeholders—including academies around the world—is important in this effort. She recalled that during her time as health commissioner in New York City in the 1990s, a resurgence of TB included unexpected and unwelcome drug resistance. This issue was successfully addressed because there was a plan that identified critical goals and objectives and involved stakeholders from different sectors, disciplines, and public and private organizations across the city. The Department of Health helped stakeholders understand the nature and scope of the problem, the strategies needed to address it, and their specific roles and responsibilities in the effort. All parties involved were held accountable for progress. Hamburg noted that this approach is challenging in a city the size of New York, much less on a global stage, even though the same issues apply.

Castro emphasized a well-known adage: Never let a crisis go to waste. He stated that the COVID-19 pandemic has provided such a crisis, noting that many speakers in this workshop have highlighted the need and ways to leverage and align the work in the TB field to bolster future PPR. He closed with optimism that the energy evident throughout the workshop would be channeled toward eliminating TB.

---

[10] This is an umbrella organization that consists of academies of science and medicine around the world. See https://www.interacademies.org (accessed January 2, 2022).

Appendix A

References

Ahmed, A., S. Rakshit, V. Adiga, M. Dias, P. Dwarkanath, G. D'Souza, and A. Vyakarnam. 2021. A century of BCG: Impact on tuberculosis control and beyond. *Immunol Rev* 301:98-121.

Aldridge, B. B., D. Barros-Aguirre, C. E. Barry 3rd, R. H. Bates, S. J. Berthel, H. I. Boshoff, K. Chibale, X. J. Chu, C. B. Cooper, V. Dartois, K. Duncan, N. Fotouhi, F. Gusovsky, P. A. Hipskind, D. J. Kempf, J. Lelievre, A. J. Lenaerts, C. W. McNamara, V. Mizrahi, C. Nathan, D. B. Olsen, T. Parish, H. M. Petrassi, A. Pym, K. Y. Rhee, G. T. Robertson, J. M. Rock, E. J. Rubin, B. Russell, D. G. Russell, J. C. Sacchettini, D. Schnappinger, M. Schrimpf, A. M. Upton, P. Warner, P. G. Wyatt, and Y. Yuan. 2021. The tuberculosis drug accelerator at year 10: What have we learned? *Nat Med* 27(8):1333-1337.

Al-Khatib, S. M., N. M. A. Lapointe, J. M. Kramer, and R. M. Califf. 2003. What clinicians should know about the QT interval. *JAMA* 289(16).

Aronson, J. D., and C. F. Aronson. 1952. Appraisal of protective value of BCG vaccine. *JAMA* 149(4):334-343.

Aronson, N. E., M. Santosham, G. W. Comstock, R. S. Howard, L. H. Moulton, E. R. Rhoades, and L. H. Harrison. 2004. Long-term efficacy of BCG vaccine in American Indians and Alaska natives: A 60-year follow-up study. *JAMA* 291(17):2086-2091.

Banco, E. 2021. Inside America's COVID-reporting breakdown. *Politico*, August 15.

Barreto, M. L., L. C. Rodrigues, S. S. Cunha, S. Pereira, M. A. Hijjar, M. Y. Ichihara, S. C. de Brito, and I. Dourado. 2002. Design of the Brazilian BCG-REVAC trial against tuberculosis: A large, simple randomized community trial to evaluate the impact on tuberculosis of BCG revaccination at school age. *Control Clin Trials* 23(5):540-553.

Barreto, M. L., S. M. Pereira, D. Pilger, A. A. Cruz, S. S. Cunha, C. Sant'Anna, M. Y. Ichihara, B. Genser, and L. C. Rodrigues. 2011. Evidence of an effect of BCG revaccination on incidence of tuberculosis in school-aged children in Brazil: Second report of the BCG-REVAC cluster-randomised trial. *Vaccine* 29(31):4875-4877.

Bernard, K. W. 2013. Health and national security: A contemporary collision of cultures. *Biosecur Bioterror* 11(2):157-162.

Bloom, B. R., and C. J. Murray. 1992. Tuberculosis: Commentary on a reemergent killer. *Science* 257(5073):1055-1064.

Bloom, K., F. van den Berg, and P. Arbuthnot. 2021. Self-amplifying RNA vaccines for infectious diseases. *Gene Ther* 28(3-4):117-129.

Bosch, B., M. A. DeJesus, N. C. Poulton, W. Zhang, C. A. Engelhart, A. Zaveri, S. Lavalette, N. Ruecker, C. Trujillo, J. B. Wallach, S. Li, S. Ehrt, B. T. Chait, D. Schnappinger, and J. M. Rock. 2021. Genome-wide gene expression tuning reveals diverse vulnerabilities of *M. tuberculosis*. *Cell* 184(17):4579-4592.e4524.

Boyce, M. R., A. Attal-Juncqua, J. Lin, S. McKay, and R. Katz. 2021. Global fund contributions to health security in ten countries, 2014-20: Mapping synergies between vertical disease programmes and capacities for preventing, detecting, and responding to public health emergencies. *Lancet Glob Health* 9(2):e181-e188.

Branigan, D. 2020. Advancing access through market interventions: Lessons learned from the GeneXpert tuberculosis test buy-down. Treatment Action Group. September. https://www.treatmentactiongroup.org/wp-content/uploads/2020/09/tag_geneXpert_lessons_learned_brief_final.pdf (accessed September 5, 2021).

Brazier, B., and H. McShane. 2020. Towards new TB vaccines. *Semin Immunopathol* 42(3):315-331.

Brito, L. A., M. Chan, C. A. Shaw, A. Hekele, T. Carsillo, M. Schaefer, J. Archer, A. Seubert, G. R. Otten, C. W. Beard, A. K. Dey, A. Lilja, N. M. Valiante, P. W. Mason, C. W. Mandl, S. W. Barnett, P. R. Dormitzer, J. B. Ulmer, M. Singh, D. T. O'Hagan, and A. J. Geall. 2014. A cationic nanoemulsion for the delivery of next-generation RNA vaccines. *Mol Ther* 22(12):2118-2129.

Budd, J., B. S. Miller, E. M. Manning, V. Lampos, M. Zhuang, M. Edelstein, G. Rees, V. C. Emery, M. M. Stevens, N. Keegan, M. J. Short, D. Pillay, E. Manley, I. J. Cox, D. Heymann, A. M. Johnson, and R. A. McKendry. 2020. Digital technologies in the public-health response to COVID-19. *Nat Med* 26(8):1183-1192.

Cadena, A. M., J. L. Flynn, and S. M. Fortune. 2016. The importance of first impressions: Early events in *Mycobacterium tuberculosis* infection influence outcome. *MBio* 7(2):e00342-00316.

CDC (Centers for Disease Control and Prevention). 2014. *The difference between latent TB infection and TB disease*. https://www.cdc.gov/tb/publications/factsheets/general/ltbiandactivetb.htm (accessed February 7, 2022).

CDC. 2020. *Landmark TB trial identifies shorter-course treatment regimen*. https://www.cdc.gov/nchhstp/newsroom/2020/landmark-tb-trial-media-statement.html (accessed June 29, 2022).

Celine, V., and L. Yuanqing. 2014. A comparative review of toll-like receptor 4 expression and functionality in different animal species. *Front Immunol* 5. doi:10.3389/fimmu.2014.00316.

Cheney, C. 2021. Consensus or chaos? Pandemic response hinges on trust, experts say. *Devex*, January 22.

Chihota, V., Z. Waggie, V. Cardenas, N. Martinson, G. Yimer, A. L. Garcia-Basteiro, S. van den Hof, R. E. Chaisson, K. L Fielding, and G. Churchyard. 2021. Safety of short-course weekly rifapentine and isoniazid (3HP) for TB preventive treatment during pregnancy (abstract). *Int J Tuberc Lung Dis* 25(10, Supp 2):S61-S62.

Cilloni, L., H. Fu, J. F. Vesga, D. Dowdy, C. Pretorius, S. Ahmedov, S. A. Nair, A. Mosneaga, E. Masini, S. Sahu, and N. Arinaminpathy. 2020. The potential impact of the COVID-19 pandemic on the tuberculosis epidemic a modelling analysis. *EClinicalMedicine* 28:100603.

Codlin, A. J., T. P. Dao, L. N. Q. Vo, R. J. Forse, V. V. Truong, H. M. Dang, L. H. Nguyen, H. B. Nguyen, N. V. Nguyen, K. Sidney-Annerstedt, B. Squire, K. Lönnroth, and M. Caws. 2021. Independent evaluation of 12 artificial intelligence solutions for the detection of tuberculosis. *Sci Rep* 11:23895.

Coleman, C. N., M. K. Mansoura, M. J. Marinissen, S. Grover, M. Dosanjh, H. D. Brereton, L. Roth, E. Wendling, D. A. Pistenmaa, and D. M. O'Brien. 2020. Achieving flexible competence: Bridging the investment dichotomy between infectious diseases and cancer. *BMJ Glob Health* 5(12):e003252.

Coler, R. N., S. Bertholet, S. O. Pine, M. T. Orr, V. Reese, H. P. Windish, C. Davis, M. Kahn, S. L. Baldwin, and S. G. Reed. 2013. Therapeutic immunization against *Mycobacterium tuberculosis* is an effective adjunct to antibiotic treatment. *J Infect Dis* 207(8):1242-1252.

Comstock, G. W., and C. E. Palmer. 1966. Long-term results of BCG vaccination in the southern United States. *Am Rev Respir Dis* 93(2):171-183.

Connolly, L. E., P. H. Edelstein, and L. Ramakrishnan. 2007. Why is long-term therapy required to cure tuberculosis? *PLoS Med* 4(3):e120. https://doi.org/10.1371/journal.pmed.0040120.

Crosby, S., J. L. Dieleman, S. Kiernan, and T. J. Bollyky. 2020. All bets are off for measuring pandemic preparedness. *Think Global Health*, June 30.

Cutler, D. M., and L. H. Summers. 2020. The COVID-19 pandemic and the $16 trillion virus. *JAMA* 324(15):1495-1496.

Denayer, T., T. Stöhrn, and M. Van Roy. 2014. Animal models in translational medicine: Validation and prediction. *New Horiz Transl Med* 2(1):5-11.

Dooley, K. E., R. Savic, A. Gupte, M. A. Marzinke, N. Zhang, V. A. Edward, L. Wolf, M. Sebe, M. Likoti, M. J. Fyvie, I. Shibambo, T. Beattie, R. E. Chaisson, G. J. Churchyard, and D. S. Team. 2020. Once-weekly rifapentine and isoniazid for tuberculosis prevention in patients with HIV taking dolutegravir-based antiretroviral therapy: A phase 1/2 trial. *Lancet HIV* 7(6):e401-e409.

Dorman, S. E., P. Nahid, E. V. Kurbatova, S. V. Goldberg, L. Bozeman, W. J. Burman, K. C. Chang, M. Chen, M. Cotton, K. E. Dooley, M. Engle, P. J. Feng, C. V. Fletcher, P. Ha, C. M. Heilig, J. L. Johnson, E. Lessem, B. Metchock, J. M. Miro, N. V. Nhung, A. C. Pettit, P. P. J. Phillips, A. T. Podany, A. E. Purfield, K. Robergeau, W. Samaneka, N. A. Scott, E. Sizemore, A. Vernon, M. Weiner, S. Swindells, and R. E. Chaisson. 2020. High-dose rifapentine with or without moxifloxacin for shortening treatment of pulmonary tuberculosis: Study protocol for TBTC study 31/ACTGa5349 phase 3 clinical trial. *Contemp Clin Trials* 90:105938.

Dorman, S. E., P. Nahid, E. V. Kurbatova, P. P. J. Phillips, K. Bryant, K. E. Dooley, M. Engle, S. V. Goldberg, H. T. T. Phan, J. Hakim, J. L. Johnson, M. Lourens, N. A. Martinson, G. Muzanyi, K. Narunsky, S. Nerette, N. V. Nguyen, T. H. Pham, S. Pierre, A. E. Purfield, W. Samaneka, R. M. Savic, I. Sanne, N. A. Scott, J. Shenje, E. Sizemore, A. Vernon, Z. Waja, M. Weiner, S. Swindells, R. E. Chaisson, A. C. T. Group, and C. Tuberculosis Trials. 2021. Four-month rifapentine regimens with or without moxifloxacin for tuberculosis. *N Engl J Med* 384(18):1705-1718.

Eregata, G. T., A. Hailu, K. Stenberg, K. A. Johansson, O. F. Norheim, and M. Y. Bertram. 2021. Generalised cost-effectiveness analysis of 159 health interventions for the Ethiopian essential health service package. *Cost Eff Resour Alloc* 19(1):2.

Ernest, J. P., N. Strydom, Q. Wang, N. Zhang, E. Nuermberger, V. Dartois, and R. M. Savic. 2021. Development of new tuberculosis drugs: Translation to regimen composition for drug-sensitive and multidrug-resistant tuberculosis. *Annu Rev Pharmacol Toxicol* 61:495-516.

Fourth Report (Fourth Report to the Medical Research Council by Its Tuberculosis Vaccines Clinical Trials Committee). 1972. BCG and vole bacillus vaccines in the prevention of tuberculosis in adolescence and early adult life. *Bull World Health Organ* 46(3):371-385.

Fu, H., J. A. Lewnard, I. Frost, R. Laxminarayan, and N. Arinaminpathy. 2021. Modelling the global burden of drug-resistant tuberculosis avertable by a post-exposure vaccine. *Nat Commun* 12(1):424.

G20 HLIP (High-Level Independent Panel on Financing the Global Commons for Pandemic Preparedness and Response). 2021. *A global deal for our pandemic age*. https://www.bruegel.org/2021/07/a-global-deal-for-our-pandemic-age (accessed February 28, 2022).

Garçon, N., and A. Di Pasquale. 2017. From discovery to licensure, the Adjuvant System story. *Hum Vaccin Immunother* 13(1):19-33.

Geske, D. 2021. Nearly 17M Americans may have went undiagnosed with covid last year: Why these cases matter. *International Business Times*, June.

Global Fund (Global Fund to Fight AIDS, Tuberculosis and Malaria). 2021. *Results report 2021*. Geneva, Switzerland: The Global Fund to Fight AIDS, Tuberculosis and Malaria.

Global TB Caucus. 2017. *The price of a pandemic*. https://www.tbonline.info/posts/2017/11/26/price-pandemic-2017 (accessed February 24, 2022).

Golub, J. E., C. I. Mohan, G. W. Comstock, and R. E. Chaisson. 2005. Active case finding of tuberculosis: Historical perspective and future prospects. *Int J Tuberc Lung Dis* 9(11):1183-1203.

Gorvett, Z. 2021. The race to understand "immune amnesia." *BBC Future*. November 15.

Gupta, A., S. Swindells, S. Kim, M. D. Hughes, L. Naini, X. Wu, R. Dawson, V. Mave, J. Sanchez, and A. Mendoza. 2020. Feasibility of identifying household contacts of rifampin- and multidrug-resistant tuberculosis cases at high risk of progression to tuberculosis disease. *Clin Infect Dis* 70(3):425-435.

Hackett, M. 2020. Average cost of hospital care for COVID-19 ranges from $51,000 to $78,000, based on age. Healthcare Finance. November 5. https://www.healthcarefinancenews.com/news/average-cost-hospital-care-covid-19-ranges-51000-78000-based-age (accessed January 5, 2022).

Heimbeck, J. 1948. BCG vaccination of nurses. *Tubercle* 29(4):84-88.

Imperial, M. Z., P. Nahid, P. P. J. Phillips, G. R. Davies, K. Fielding, D. Hanna, D. Hermann, R. S. Wallis, J. L. Johnson, C. Lienhardt, and R. M. Savic. 2018. A patient-level pooled analysis of treatment-shortening regimens for drug-susceptible pulmonary tuberculosis. *Nat Med* 24(11):1708-1715.

IOM (Institute of Medicine). 2011. *The new profile of drug-resistant tuberculosis in Russia: A global and local perspective: Summary of a joint workshop by the Institute of Medicine and the Russian Academy of Medical Science*. Washington, DC: The National Academies Press. https://doi.org/10.17226/13033 (accessed February 24, 2022).

IOM. 2012. *Facing the reality of drug-resistant tuberculosis in India: Challenges and potential solutions: Summary of a joint workshop by the Institute of Medicine, the Indian National Science Academy, and the Indian Council of Medical Research*. Washington, DC: The National Academies Press.

IOM. 2014. *The global crisis of drug-resistant tuberculosis and leadership of China and the BRICS: Challenges and opportunities: Summary of a joint workshop by the Institute of Medicine and the Institute of Microbiology, Chinese Academy of Sciences*. Washington, DC: The National Academies Press. https://doi.org/10.17226/18346 (accessed February 24, 2022).

Jamison, D. T., L. H. Summers, G. Alleyne, K. J. Arrow, S. Berkley, A. Binagwaho, F. Bustreo, D. Evans, R. G. A. Feachem, J. Frenk, G. Ghosh, S. J. Goldie, Y. Guo, S. Gupta, R. Horton, M. E. Kruk, A. Mahmoud, L. K. Mohohlo, M. Ncube, A. Pablos-Mendez, K. S. Reddy, H. Saxenian, A. Soucat, K. H. Ulltveit-Moe, and G. Yamey. 2013. Global health 2035: A world converging within a generation. *Lancet* 382(9908):1898-1955.

Joung, J., A. Ladha, M. Saito, N. G. Kim, A. E. Woolley, M. Segel, R. P. J. Barretto, A. Ranu, R. K. Macrae, G. Faure, E. I. Ioannidi, R. N. Krajeski, R. Bruneau, M. W. Huang, X. G. Yu, J. Z. Li, B. D. Walker, D. T. Hung, A. L. Greninger, K. R. Jerome, J. S. Gootenberg, O. O. Abudayyeh, and F. Zhang. 2020. Detection of SARS-CoV-2 with Sherlock one-pot testing. *N Engl J Med* 383(15):1492-1494.

Kaplan, G. J., R. I. Fraser, and G. W. Comstock. 1972. Tuberculosis in Alaska, 1970. The continued decline of the tuberculosis epidemic. *Am Rev Respir Dis* 105(6):920-926.

Karonga Prevention Trial Group. Randomised controlled trial of single BCG, repeated BCG, or combined BCG and killed *Mycobacterium leprae* vaccine for prevention of leprosy and tuberculosis in Malawi. 1996. *Lancet* 348(9019):17-24.

Kasaie, P., J. R. Andrews, W. D. Kelton, and D. W. Dowdy. 2014. Timing of tuberculosis transmission and the impact of household contact tracing. An agent-based simulation model. *Am J Respir Crit Care Med* 189(7):845-852.

Katz, R., and A. Vaught. 2017. Controlling tuberculosis in the United States: Use of isolation and other measures throughout the country. *Disaster Med Public Health Prep* 11(3):337-342.

Keshavjee, S., I. Y. Gelmanova, A. D. Pasechnikov, S. P. Mishustin, Y. G. Andreev, A. Yedilbayev, J. J. Furin, J. S. Mukherjee, M. L. Rich, E. A. Nardell, P. E. Farmer, J. Y. Kim, and S. S. Shin. 2008. Treating multidrug-resistant tuberculosis in Tomsk, Russia: Developing programs that address the linkage between poverty and disease. *Ann NY Acad Sci* 1136:1-11.

Korbee, C. J., M. T. Heemskerk, D. Kocev, E. van Strijen, O. Rabiee, K. L. Franken, L. Wilson, N. D. Savage, S. Džeroski, and M. C. Haks. 2018. Combined chemical genetics and data-driven bioinformatics approach identifies receptor tyrosine kinase inhibitors as host-directed antimicrobials. *Nat Commun* 9(1):1-14.

Kyu, H. H., E. R. Maddison, N. J. Henry, J. R. Ledesma, K. E. Wiens, R. Reiner, M. H. Biehl, C. Shields, A. Osgood-Zimmerman, J. M. Ross, A. Carter, T. D. Frank, H. Wang, V. Srinivasan, S. K. Agarwal, F. Alahdab, K. A. Alene, B. A. Ali, N. Alvis-Guzman, J. R. Andrews, C. A. T. Antonio, S. Atique, S. R. Atre, A. Awasthi, H. T. Ayele, H. Badali, A. Badawi, A. Barac, N. Bedi, M. Behzadifar, B. B. Bekele, S. A. Belay, I. M. Bensenor, Z. A. Butt, F. Carvalho, K. Cercy, D. J. Christopher, A. K. Daba, L. Dandona, R. Dandona, A. Daryani, F. M. Demeke, K. Deribe, S. D. Dharmaratne, D. T. Doku, M. Dubey, D. Edessa, Z. El-Khatib, S. Enany, E. Fernandes, F. Fischer, A. L. Garcia-Basteiro, A. K. Gebre, G. B. Gebregergs, T. G. Gebremichael, T. F. Gelano, D. Geremew, P. N. Gona, A. Goodridge, R. Gupta, H. Haghparast Bidgoli, G. B. Hailu, H. Y. Hassen, M. T. T. Hedayati, A. Henok, S. Hostiuc, M. A. Hussen, O. S. Ilesanmi, S. S. N. Irvani, K. H. Jacobsen, S. C. Johnson, J. B. Jonas, A. Kahsay, S. Kant, A. Kasaeian, T. D. Kassa, Y. S. Khader, M. A. Khafaie, I. Khalil, E. A. Khan, Y.-H. Khang, Y. J. Kim, S. Kochhar, A. Koyanagi, K. J. Krohn, G. A. Kumar, A. M. Lakew, C. T. Leshargie, R. Lodha, E. R. K. Macarayan, R. Majdzadeh, F. R. Martins-Melo, A. Melese, Z. A. Memish, W. Mendoza, D. T. Mengistu, G. Mengistu, T. Mestrovic, B. Moazen, K. A. Mohammad, S. Mohammed, A. H. Mokdad, M. Moosazadeh, S. M. Mousavi, G. Mustafa, J. B. Nachega, T. H. Nguyen, S. H. Nguyen, T. H. Nguyen, D. N. A. Ningrum, Y. L. Nirayo, V. M. Nong, R. Ofori-Asenso, F. A. Ogbo, I.-H. Oh, O. Oladimeji, A. T. Olagunju, E. Oren, D. M. Pereira, S. Prakash, M. Qorbani, A. Rafay, R. K. Rai, U. Ram, S. Rubino, S. Safiri, J. A. Salomon, A. M. Samy, B. Sartorius, M. Satpathy, S. Seyedmousavi, M. Sharif, J. P. Silva, D. G. A. Silveira, J. A. Singh, C. T. Sreeramareddy, B. X. Tran, A. G. Tsadik, K. N. Ukwaja, I. Ullah, O. A. Uthman, V. Vlassov, S. E. Vollset, G. Vu, F. Weldegebreal, A. Werdecker, E. M. Yimer, N. Yonemoto, M. Yotebieng, M. Naghavi, T. Vos, S. I. Hay, and C. J. L. Murray. 2018. Global, regional, and national burden of tuberculosis, 1990–2016: Results from the global burden of diseases, injuries, and risk factors 2016 study. *Lancet Infect Dis* 18(12):1329-1349.

Lakshminarayana, S. B., T. B. Huat, P. C. Ho, U. H. Manjunatha, V. Dartois, T. Dick, and S. P. Rao. 2015. Comprehensive physicochemical, pharmacokinetic and activity profiling of anti-TB agents. *J Antimicrob Chemother* 70(3):857-867.

Lienhardt, C., and P. Nahid. 2019. Advances in clinical trial design for development of new TB treatments: A call for innovation. *PLoS Med* 16(3):e1002769.

Lomborg, B. 2015. *The Nobel laureates guide to the smartest targets for the world 2016-2030*. Tewksbury, MA: Copenhagen Consensus Center.

Lomborg, B. 2018. *Prioritizing development: A cost benefit analysis of the United Nations' Sustainable Development Goals*. Cambridge, UK: Cambridge University Press.

MacLean, E., M. Kohli, S. F. Weber, A. Suresh, S. G. Schumacher, C. M. Denkinger, and M. Pai. 2020. Advances in molecular diagnosis of tuberculosis. *J Clin Microbiol* 58(10):e01582-01519.

Malone, R. W., P. L. Felgner, and I. M. Verma. 1989. Cationic liposome-mediated RNA transfection. *Proc Natl Acad Sci USA* 86(16):6077-6081.

Menzies, N. A., M. Quaife, B. W. Allwood, A. L. Byrne, A. K. Coussens, A. D. Harries, F. M. Marx, J. Meghji, D. Pedrazzoli, J. A. Salomon, S. Sweeney, S. C. van Kampen, R. S. Wallis, R. M. G. J. Houben, and T. Cohen. 2021. Lifetime burden of disease due to incident tuberculosis: A global reappraisal including post-tuberculosis sequelae. *Lancet Glob Health* 9(12):e1679-e1687.

Miller, S. L., W. W. Nazaroff, J. L. Jimenez, A. Boerstra, G. Buonanno, S. J. Dancer, J. Kurnitski, L. C. Marr, L. Morawska, and C. Noakes. 2021. Transmission of SARS-CoV-2 by inhalation of respiratory aerosol in the Skagit Valley Chorale superspreading event. *Indoor Air* 31(2):314-323.

Milton, D. 2020. A Rosetta Stone for understanding infectious drops and aerosols. *J Pediatric Infect Dis Soc* 9(4):413-415.

Mphaphlele, M., A. S. Dharmadhikari, P. A. Jensen, S. N. Rudnick, T. H. van Reenen, M. A. Pagano, W. Leuschner, T. A. Sears, S. P. Milonova, M. van der Walt, A. C. Stoltz, K. Weyer, and E. A. Nardell. 2015. Institutional tuberculosis transmission. Controlled trial of upper room ultraviolet air disinfection: A basis for new dosing guidelines. *Am J Respir Crit Care Med* 192(4):477-484.

Nakajima, H. 1993. Tuberculosis: A global emergency. *World Health* 46(4):3-3.

Napier, R. J., W. Rafi, M. Cheruvu, K. R. Powell, M. A. Zaunbrecher, W. Bornmann, P. Salgame, T. M. Shinnick, and D. Kalman. 2011. Imatinib-sensitive tyrosine kinases regulate mycobacterial pathogenesis and represent therapeutic targets against tuberculosis. *Cell Host Microbe* 10(5):475-485.

Napier, R. J., B. A. Norris, A. Swimm, C. R. Giver, W. A. Harris, J. Laval, B. A. Napier, G. Patel, R. Crump, Z. Peng, W. Bornmann, B. Pulendran, R. M. Buller, D. S. Weiss, R. Tirouvanziam, E. K. Waller, and D. Kalman. 2015. Low doses of imatinib induce myelopoiesis and enhance host anti-microbial immunity. *PLoS Pathog* 11(3):e1004770.

Narasimhan, P., J. Wood, C. R. MacIntyre, and D. Mathai. 2013. Risk factors for tuberculosis. *Pulm Med* 828939. https://doi.org/10.1155/2013/828939.

Nardell, E. A. 2021. Air disinfection for airborne infection control with a focus on COVID-19: Why germicidal UV is essential. *Photochem Photobiol* 97(3):493-497.

Nardell, E., P. Lederer, H. Mishra, R. Nathavitharana, and G. Theron. 2020. Cool but dangerous: How climate change is increasing the risk of airborne infections. *Indoor Air* 30(2):195.

Ndjeka, N., J. Hughes, A. Reuter, F. Conradie, M. Enwerem, H. Ferreira, N. Ismail, Y. Kock, I. Master, G. Meintjes, X. Padanilam, R. Romero, H. S. Schaaf, J. T. Riele, and G. Maartens. 2020. Implementing novel regimens for drug-resistant TB in South Africa: What can the world learn? *Int J Tuberc Lung Dis* 24(10):1073-1080.

Nemes, E., H. Geldenhuys, V. Rozot, K. T. Rutkowski, F. Ratangee, N. Bilek, S. Mabwe, L. Makhethe, M. Erasmus, A. Toefy, H. Mulenga, W. A. Hanekom, S. G. Self, L. G. Bekker, R. Ryall, S. Gurunathan, C. A. DiazGranados, P. Andersen, I. Kromann, T. Evans, R. D. Ellis, B. Landry, D. A. Hokey, R. Hopkins, A. M. Ginsberg, T. J. Scriba, M. Hatherill, and C. S. Team. 2018. Prevention of M. tuberculosis infection with h4:Ic31 vaccine or BCG revaccination. *N Engl J Med* 379(2):138-149.

Otu, A. A. 2013. Is the Directly Observed Therapy Short Course (DOTS) an effective strategy for tuberculosis control in a developing country? *Asian Pacific J Trop Dis* 3(3):227-231.

Outterson, K., E. S. F. Orubu, J. Rex, C. Årdal, and M. H. Zaman. 2022. Patient access in 14 high-income countries to new antibacterials approved by the US Food and Drug Administration, European Medicines Agency, Japanese Pharmaceuticals and Medical Devices Agency, or Health Canada, 2010–2020. *Clin Infect Dis* 74(7):1183-1190.

Oxlade, O., S. den Boon, D. Menzies, D. Falzon, M. Y. Lane, A. Kanchar, M. Zignol, and A. Matteelli. 2021. TB preventive treatment in high- and intermediate-incidence countries: Research needs for scale-up. *Int J Tuberc Lung Dis* 25(10):823-831.

Paget, C., and F. Trottein. 2019. Mechanisms of bacterial superinfection post-influenza: A role for unconventional T cells. *Front Immunol* 10. https://doi.org/10.3389/fimmu.2019.00336.

Partners In Health. 2006. *New guidelines and goals for treating MDR-TB announced.* https://www.pih.org/article/new-guidelines-and-goals-for-treating-mdr-tb-announced (accessed February 2, 2022).

Polack, F. P., S. J. Thomas, N. Kitchin, J. Absalon, A. Gurtman, S. Lockhart, J. L. Perez, G. Perez Marc, E. D. Moreira, C. Zerbini, R. Bailey, K. A. Swanson, S. Roychoudhury, K. Koury, P. Li, W. V. Kalina, D. Cooper, R. W. Frenck Jr., L. L. Hammitt, O. Tureci, H. Nell, A. Schaefer, S. Unal, D. B. Tresnan, S. Mather, P. R. Dormitzer, U. Sahin, K. U. Jansen, W. C. Gruber, and C. C. T. Group. 2020. Safety and efficacy of the BNT162b2 mRNA COVID-19 vaccine. *N Engl J Med* 383(27):2603-2615.

Reid, M., and G. Yamey. 2019. A roadmap for ending the moral catastrophe of TB. *Global Health Now*, March 20. https://www.globalhealthnow.org/2019-03/roadmap-ending-moral-catastrophe-tb (accessed September 14, 2021).

Reid, M. J. A., N. Arinaminpathy, A. Bloom, B. R. Bloom, C. Boehme, R. Chaisson, D. P. Chin, G. Churchyard, H. Cox, L. Ditiu, M. Dybul, J. Farrar, A. S. Fauci, E. Fekadu, P. I. Fujiwara, T. B. Hallett, C. L. Hanson, M. Harrington, N. Herbert, P. C. Hopewell, C. Ikeda, D. T. Jamison, A. J. Khan, I. Koek, N. Krishnan, A. Motsoaledi, M. Pai, M. C. Raviglione, A. Sharman, P. M. Small, S. Swaminathan, Z. Temesgen, A. Vassall, N. Venkatesan, K. van Weezenbeek, G. Yamey, B. D. Agins, S. Alexandru, J. R. Andrews, N. Beyeler, S. Bivol, G. Brigden, A. Cattamanchi, D. Cazabon, V. Crudu, A. Daftary, P. Dewan, L. K. Doepel, R. W. Eisinger, V. Fan, S. Fewer, J. Furin, J. D. Goldhaber-Fiebert, G. B. Gomez, S. M. Graham, D. Gupta, M. Kamene, S. Khaparde, E. W. Mailu, E. O. Masini, L. McHugh, E. Mitchell, S. Moon, M. Osberg, T. Pande, L. Prince, K. Rade, R. Rao, M. Remme, J. A. Seddon, C. Selwyn, P. Shete, K. S. Sachdeva, G. Stallworthy, J. F. Vesga, V. Vilc, and E. P. Goosby. 2019. Building a tuberculosis-free world: The Lancet Commission on Tuberculosis. *Lancet* 393(10178):1331-1384.

Reid, M. J. A., S. Silva, N. Arinaminpathy, and E. Goosby. 2020. Building a tuberculosis-free world while responding to the COVID-19 pandemic. *Lancet* 396(10259):1312-1313.

Rueckert, C., and C. A. Guzmán. 2012. Vaccines: From empirical development to rational design. *PLoS Pathog* 8(11):e1003001.

Ruhwald, M., S. Carmona, and M. Pai. 2021. Learning from COVID-19 to reimagine tuberculosis diagnosis. *Lancet Microbe* 2(5):e169-e170.

Sabin, L. L., M. B. DeSilva, D. H. Hamer, K. Xu, J. Zhang, T. Li, I. B. Wilson, and C. J. Gill. 2010. Using electronic drug monitor feedback to improve adherence to antiretroviral therapy among HIV-positive patients in China. *AIDS Behav* 14(3):580-589.

Sharma, A., A. Hill, E. Kurbatova, M. van der Walt, C. Kvasnovsky, T. E. Tupasi, J. C. Caoili, M. T. Gler, G. V. Volchenkov, B. Y. Kazennyy, O. V. Demikhova, J. Bayona, C. Contreras, M. Yagui, V. Leimane, S. N. Cho, H. J. Kim, K. Kliiman, S. Akksilp, R. Jou, J. Ershova, T. Dalton, P. Cegielski, and Global Preserving Effective TB Treatment Study Investigators. 2017. Estimating the future burden of multidrug-resistant and extensively drug-resistant tuberculosis in India, the Philippines, Russia, and South Africa: A mathematical modelling study. *Lancet Infect Dis* 17(7):707-715.

Silva, S., N. Arinaminpathy, R. Atun, E. Goosby, and M. Reid. 2021. Economic impact of tuberculosis mortality in 120 countries and the cost of not achieving the Sustainable Development Goals tuberculosis targets: A full-income analysis. *Lancet Glob Health* 9(10):e1372-e1379.

Stop TB Partnership. 2020. *The potential impact of the COVID-19 response on tuberculosis in high-burden countries: A modelling analysis.* https://stoptb.org/assets/documents/news/Modeling%20Report_1%20May%202020_FINAL.pdf (accessed February 24, 2022).

Stop TB Partnership. 2021. *The impact of COVID-19 on the TB epidemic: A community perspective.* https://www.stoptb.org/impact-of-covid-19-tb-epidemic-community-perspective (accessed February 24, 2022).

Stylianou, E., M. J. Paul, R. Reljic, and H. McShane. 2019. Mucosal delivery of tuberculosis vaccines: A review of current approaches and challenges. *Expert Rev Vaccines* 18(12):1271-1284.

Subbaraman, R., R. R. Nathavitharana, S. Satyanarayana, M. Pai, B. E. Thomas, V. K. Chadha, K. Rade, S. Swaminathan, and K. H. Mayer. 2016. The tuberculosis cascade of care in India's public sector: A systematic review and meta-analysis. *PLoS Med* 13(10):e1002149.

Subbaraman, R., L. de Mondesert, A. Musiimenta, M. Pai, K. H. Mayer, B. E. Thomas, and J. Haberer. 2018. Digital adherence technologies for the management of tuberculosis therapy: Mapping the landscape and research priorities. *BMJ Glob Health* 3(5):e001018.

Swindells, S., R. Ramchandani, A. Gupta, C. A. Benson, J. Leon-Cruz, N. Mwelase, M. A. Jean Juste, J. R. Lama, J. Valencia, A. Omoz-Oarhe, K. Supparatpinyo, G. Masheto, L. Mohapi, R. O. da Silva Escada, S. Mawlana, P. Banda, P. Severe, J. Hakim, C. Kanyama, D. Langat, L. Moran, J. Andersen, C. V. Fletcher, E. Nuermberger, R. E. Chaisson, and the B. T. A. S. Team. 2019. One month of rifapentine plus isoniazid to prevent HIV-related tuberculosis. *N Engl J Med* 380(11):1001-1011.

Tait, D. R., M. Hatherill, O. Van Der Meeren, A. M. Ginsberg, E. Van Brakel, B. Salaun, T. J. Scriba, E. J. Akite, H. M. Ayles, A. Bollaerts, M. A. Demoitie, A. Diacon, T. G. Evans, P. Gillard, E. Hellstrom, J. C. Innes, M. Lempicki, M. Malahleha, N. Martinson, D. Mesia Vela, M. Muyoyeta, V. Nduba, T. G. Pascal, M. Tameris, F. Thienemann, R. J. Wilkinson, and F. Roman. 2019. Final analysis of a trial of M72/AS01$_E$ vaccine to prevent tuberculosis. *N Engl J Med* 381(25):2429-2439.

TB Alliance. 2022. *STAND.* https://www.tballiance.org/portfolio/trial/5091 (accessed March 1, 2022).

TB DIAH (TB Data, Impact Assessment, and Communications Hub). 2021. *Navigating tuberculosis indicators: A guide for TB programs.* Chapel Hill, NC: TB DIAH, University of North Carolina.

Thomas, A., P. Gopi, T. Santha, V. Chandrasekaran, R. Subramani, N. Selvakumar, S. Eusuff, K. Sadacharam, and P. Narayanan. 2005. Predictors of relapse among pulmonary tuberculosis patients treated in a DOTS programme in south India. *Int Tuberc Lung Dis* 9(5):556-561.

UN (United Nations). 2018. *Political declaration of the UN General Assembly High-Level Meeting on the Fight Against Tuberculosis.* New York: UN.

Uplekar, M., S. Atre, W. A. Wells, D. Weil, R. Lopez, G. B. Migliori, and M. Raviglione. 2016. Mandatory tuberculosis case notification in high tuberculosis-incidence countries: Policy and practice. *Eur Respir J* 48(6):1571-1581.

Van Der Meeren, O., M. Hatherill, V. Nduba, R. J. Wilkinson, M. Muyoyeta, E. Van Brakel, H. M. Ayles, G. Henostroza, F. Thienemann, T. J. Scriba, A. Diacon, G. L. Blatner, M. A. Demoitie, M. Tameris, M. Malahleha, J. C. Innes, E. Hellstrom, N. Martinson, T. Singh, E. J. Akite, A. Khatoon Azam, A. Bollaerts, A. M. Ginsberg, T. G. Evans, P. Gillard, and D. R. Tait. 2018. Phase 2b controlled trial of M72/AS01$_E$ vaccine to prevent tuberculosis. *N Engl J Med* 379(17):1621-1634.

Venkatesan, P. 2020. COVID-19 diagnostics—not at the expense of other diseases. *Lancet Microbe* 1(2):e64.

Verguet, S., C. Riumallo-Herl, G. B. Gomez, N. A. Menzies, R. Houben, T. Sumner, M. Lalli, R. G. White, J. A. Salomon, T. Cohen, N. Foster, S. Chatterjee, S. Sweeney, I. G. Baena, K. Lonnroth, D. E. Weil, and A. Vassall. 2017. Catastrophic costs potentially averted by tuberculosis control in India and South Africa: A modelling study. *Lancet Glob Health* 5(11):e1123-e1132.

Vigdor, N. 2021. Months into the pandemic, the U.S. had six times as many cases as reported, an N.I.H. study finds. *New York Times*, June 24.

Vo, L. N. Q., A. Codlin, T. D. Ngo, T. P. Dao, T. T. T. Dong, H. T. L. Mo, R. Forse, T. T. Nguyen, C. V. Cung, H. B. Nguyen, N. V. Nguyen, V. V. Nguyen, N. T. Tran, G. H. Nguyen, Z. Z. Qin, and J. Creswell. 2021. Early evaluation of an ultra-portable x-ray system for tuberculosis active case finding. *Trop Med Infect Dis* 6(3):163.

Walter, N. D., S. E. M. Born, G. T. Robertson, M. Reichlen, C. Dide-Agossou, V. A. Ektnitphong, K. Rossmassler, M. E. Ramey, A. A. Bauman, V. Ozols, S. C. Bearrows, G. Schoolnik, G. Dolganov, B. Garcia, E. Musisi, W. Worodria, L. Huang, J. L. Davis, N. V. Nguyen, H. V. Nguyen, A. T. V. Nguyen, H. Phan, C. Wilusz, B. K. Podell, N. D. Sanoussi, B. C. de Jong, C. S. Merle, D. Affolabi, H. McIlleron, M. Garcia-Cremades, E. Maidji, F. Eshun-Wilson, B. Aguilar-Rodriguez, D. Karthikeyan, K. Mdluli, C. Bansbach, A. J. Lenaerts, R. M. Savic, P. Nahid, J. J. Vásquez, and M. I. Voskuil. 2021. *Mycobacterium tuberculosis* precursor rRNA as a measure of treatment-shortening activity of drugs and regimens. *Nat Commun* 12(1):2899.

Wells, W., M. Wells, and T. Wilder. 1942. The environmental control of epidemic contagion. I. An epidemiologic study of radiant disinfection of air in day schools. *Am J Hyg* 35:97-121.

WHO (World Health Organization). 2011. *Early detection of tuberculosos: An overview of approaches, guidelines and tools.* Geneva, Switzerland: World Health Organization.

WHO. 2014. *WHO handbook for guideline development.* Geneva, Switzerland: World Health Organization.

WHO. 2015. *The End TB strategy.* Geneva, Switzerland: World Health Organization.

WHO. 2018. *WHO treatment guidelines for isoniazid-resistant tuberculosis.* Geneva, Switzerland: World Health Organization.

WHO. 2019. *Global tuberculosis report 2019.* Geneva, Switzerland: World Health Organization.

WHO. 2020. *Global tuberculosis report 2020.* Geneva, Switzerland: World Health Organization.

WHO. 2021a. *Catalogue of mutations in* Mycobacterium tuberculosis *complex and their association with drug resistance.* Geneva, Switzerland: World Health Organization.

WHO. 2021b. *Impact of the COVID-19 pandemic on TB detection and mortality in 2020.* Geneva, Switzerland: World Health Organization.

WHO. 2021c. *Regional strategic plan towards ending TB in the WHO South-East Asia Region: 2021-2025.* India: World Health Organization.

WHO. 2021d. *Tuberculosis.* https://www.who.int/news-room/fact-sheets/detail/tuberculosis#:~:text=Multidrug%2Dresistant%20TB%20(MDR%2D,the%20cumulative%20reduction%20was%2011%25 (accessed March 1, 2022).

Young, C., G. Walzl, and N. Du Plessis. 2020. Therapeutic host-directed strategies to improve outcome in tuberculosis. *Mucosal Immunol* 13:190-204.

Yusuf, Y., T. Yoshii, M. Iyori, K. Yoshida, H. Mizukami, S. Fukumoto, D. S. Yamamoto, A. Alam, T. B. Emran, F. Amelia, A. Islam, H. Otsuka, E. Takashima, T. Tsuboi, and S. Yoshida. 2019. Adeno-associated virus as an effective malaria booster vaccine following adenovirus priming. *Front Immunol* 10:730.

Zaretsky, A. G., J. B. Engiles, and C. A. Hunter. 2014. Infection-induced changes in hematopoiesis. *J Immunol* 192(1):27-33.

Zhang, T., S. Y. Li, K. N. Williams, K. Andries, and E. L. Nuermberger. 2011. Short-course chemotherapy with TMC207 and rifapentine in a murine model of latent tuberculosis infection. *Am J Respir Crit Care Med* 184(6):732-737.

Appendix B

Workshop Statement of Task

A planning committee of the National Academies of Sciences, Engineering, and Medicine will organize and conduct a two-part public workshop series to explore future innovations to meet the targets in the World Health Organization's End TB Strategy by 2030.

The public workshop series will feature invited presentations and discussions to explore the following questions:

- How can we accelerate the development of affordable point-of-care tests for TB? What barriers or challenges have prevented the development of accessible point-of-care tests for TB for low- and middle-income countries?
- Improvements in the usual care for TB: Can a 2-week, nontoxic treatment for drug-sensitive and drug-resistant TB be achieved?
- How can we rapidly use the TB platform, such as contact investigation, in low- to middle-income countries to address COVID-19 and other airborne infections to prevent future pandemics?
- How can we ensure increased and sustained commitments to reach the UNHLM TB targets in high-burden countries, despite the challenges from COVID-19?

The planning committee will organize the workshop series, develop the agenda, select and invite speakers and discussants, and moderate or identify moderators for the discussions. The presentations and discussions at the workshop series will be summarized in a proceedings—in brief (Part One) and a full-length proceedings (Part Two), prepared by designated *rapporteurs* in accordance with institutional guidelines.

Appendix C

Workshop Agenda

WORKSHOP PART 1
THURSDAY, JULY 22, 2021
11:00 AM–1:00 PM ET

Current State of Tuberculosis Elimination and Effect of COVID-19

11:00 AM	Welcome Remarks, Workshop Overview, and Goals **Kenneth Castro,** *workshop co-chair* **Gail Cassell,** *workshop co-chair*
11:05 AM	Opening Addresses: Current Status and Urgency of Ending TB Around the Globe **Jim Yong Kim** (Global Infrastructure Partners) **Salmaan Keshavjee** (Harvard Medical School) **Eric Rubin** (*New England Journal of Medicine*)

Challenges and Innovations
Moderator: **Lucica Ditiu**

11:30 AM	Diagnostics **Soumya Swaminathan** (World Health Organization)
11:40 AM	Vaccines and Therapeutics **Emilio Emini** (Bill & Melinda Gates Foundation)

11:50 AM	Critical Need for New Business Models **Kevin Outterson** (Boston University School of Law)
12:00 PM	*Discussion (50 min)*
12:55 PM	Wrap-up and Adjourn **Gail Cassell,** *workshop co-chair* **Kenneth Castro,** *workshop co-chair*

WORKSHOP—PART TWO
TUESDAY, SEPTEMBER 14, 2021
11:00 AM–2:30 PM ET

Workshop Opening

11:00 AM	Welcome and Workshop Goals **Peter Daszak,** *Chair, Forum on Microbial Threats, National Academy of Medicine; President, EcoHealth Alliance* **Lucica Ditiu,** *moderator, Stop TB Partnership*
11:05 AM	Sponsor Remarks **Jennifer Adams,** *Senior Deputy Assistant Administrator, Bureau for Global Health, United States Agency for International Development*
11:20 AM	Building a Tuberculosis-Free World: Progress Update **Eric Goosby** (University of California, San Francisco) *15 min Q&A* Realities of Multidrug-Resistant TB and Challenges for TB Control **Matteo Zignol** (World Health Organization) *15 min Q&A*

APPENDIX C   *169*

Session 1: Detection

12:15 PM   Rapid Acceleration of Diagnostics: The COVID-19 Experience
                  Matthew McMahon (Director, Small Business Education and Entrepreneurial Development, NIH)

                  15 min Q&A

12:45 PM   Panel Discussion on Diagnostic Advances

                  Point-of-Care Molecular Platform for Diagnosis of TB and Other Infectious Respiratory Diseases
                  Morten Ruhwald (FIND, the global alliance for diagnostics)

                  Platform Technologies for Detection of Multiple Agents
                  Zvi Marom (BATM) and **Eran Zahavy** (BATM)

                  Improving X-Ray Accessibility
                  Luan Vo (Friends for International Tuberculosis Relief)

                  Implementation Challenges with New TB Diagnostics
                  Kaiser Shen (USAID)

1:15 PM   Enhancing Adherence, Infection Control Capacities, and Cost-Effectiveness

                  Expansion and Improvements to Contact Tracing and Engagement: Mobile or Digital Platforms from the COVID-19 Pandemic
                  Aamir Khan (IRD)

                  Telehealth and Digital Adherence Technologies
                  Bruce Thomas (The Arcady Group)

                  Innovative Strategies to Share the Costs of Investments in Health Care Systems by Partnering with Other Disease Burdens in LMICs
                  Monique K. Mansoura (MITRE)

Infection Prevention
Edward Nardell (Harvard Medical School, Brigham and Women's Hospital)

Management of Latent TB Infection: Gaps and Opportunities
Gavin Churchyard (The Aurum Institute)

2:15 PM   Reflections on Session 1
Lucica Ditiu

2:30 PM   Adjourn

WORKSHOP PART 2
WEDNESDAY, SEPTEMBER 15, 2021
11:00 AM–2:30 PM ET

Session 2: Vaccines and Therapeutics

11:00 AM   Welcome and Session Goals
Kent Kester, *moderator, Sanofi Pasteur*

11:05 AM   Using Existing Tools and New Technologies

BCG Revaccination
Alex Schmidt (Bill & Melinda Gates Medical Research Institute)

Promising New Adjuvants and Late-Stage Clinical Development Vaccine Candidates
Steve Reed (University of Washington; HDT Bio)

How Host-Directed Therapies Can Change the Development Landscape
Daniel Kalman (Emory University)

Immune Mechanisms of Protection Against TB
Rhea Coler (Seattle Children's Hospital)

12:00 PM   Transforming Treatment Options
Charles Wells, *moderator, Bill & Melinda Gates Medical Research Institute*

APPENDIX C

	The Key to Success for Developing a New Regimen to Advance TB Treatment: Lessons from TBTC Study 31 (S31/A5349) **Payam Nahid** (University of California, San Francisco)
	What It Takes to Roll Out a New Treatment Regimen: Lessons from Drug-Resistant TB **Adrian Thomas** (Johnson & Johnson) **Norbert Ndjeka** (National Department of Health, Republic of South Africa)
	Bringing Innovation to the Development of New Transformative TB Regimens **David Hermann** (Bill & Melinda Gates Foundation)
	Importance of Context-Specific Economic Analyses to Inform Future Program Design and Investment **Anna Vassall** (London School of Hygiene & Tropical Medicine)
1:00 PM	Expert Reflections and Discussion on Critical Elements for Implementation **Ezra Shimeles Tessera** (TB Data, Impact Assessment and Communications Hub, USAID; John Snow, Inc.) **Richard Chaisson** (Johns Hopkins University School of Medicine and Bloomberg School of Public Health)
2:15 PM	Reflections on Session 2 **Kent Kester** **Charles Wells**
2:30 PM	Adjourn

WORKSHOP PART 2
THURSDAY, SEPTEMBER 16, 2021
11:00 AM–2:30 PM ET

Session 3: Financing, Ambition, and Preparedness

11:00 AM	Welcome: Session Goals and Bold Moves **Peter Sands**, *moderator, The Global Fund*

11:10 AM	Opening Remarks **Victor Dzau**, *President, National Academy of Medicine*
11:15 AM	A Place for TB in the Pandemic Preparedness Agenda **Tharman Shanmugaratnam**, *Senior Minister, Singapore, and co-chair, G20 High-Level Independent Panel on Financing the Global Commons for Pandemic Preparedness and Response*
11:50 AM	Achieving Synergy in Global Health Security Preparedness Against Respiratory Pathogens: Recognition of TB as a Leading Killer **Peter Sands**, *moderator* **John Bell** (University of Oxford) **Bruce Gellin** (The Rockefeller Foundation) **Rebecca Katz** (Georgetown University, Center for Global Health Science and Security) **Michael Callahan** (Massachusetts General Hospital; United Therapeutics)
1:05 PM	Making the Case for Financing TB Elimination **Margaret Hamburg**, *moderator, Nuclear Threats Initiative* The Cost of Failing to Achieve the End TB Targets: A Full Economic Analysis **Michael Reid** (University of California, San Francisco) Why TB Is One of the Best Investments on the SDG Agenda **Bjorn Lomborg** (Copenhagen Consensus Center) Smart Investments in Ending TB **Mark Dybul** (Georgetown University; Enochian BioSciences) Implications for TB from the High-Level Independent Panel on Financing the Global Commons for Pandemic Preparedness and Response **Amanda Glassman** (Center for Global Development)

2:00 PM   Closing Remarks
               Margaret Hamburg
               Gail Cassell, *workshop co-chair*
               Kenneth Castro, *workshop co-chair*

2:30 PM   Adjourn